Your Pregnancy for the
Father-to-Be

Other books by Glade B. Curtis, M.D., and Judith Schuler, M.S.

Your Pregnancy Week by Week, 4th Edition
Your Baby's First Year Week by Week
Your Pregnancy after 35, Revised Edition
Your Pregnancy Questions and Answers, 3rd Edition
Your Pregnancy: Every Woman's Guide
Your Pregnancy Journal Week by Week
Bouncing Back after Your Pregnancy

Your Pregnancy for the

Father-to-Be

❖　❖　❖

Everything Dads Need
to Know about Pregnancy,
Childbirth, and Getting
Ready for a New Baby

**Glade B. Curtis, M.D.
and Judith Schuler, M.S.**

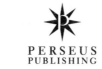

PERSEUS
PUBLISHING

A Member of the Perseus Books Group

Copyright © 2003 by Glade B. Curtis, M.D., and Judith Schuler, M.S.

Library of Congress Control Number: 2002114008
ISBN 1-55561-345-4

Perseus Publishing is a Member of the Perseus Books Group.
Find us on the World Wide Web at http://www.perseuspublishing.com.
Perseus Publishing books are available at special discounts for bulk purchases in the U.S. by corporations, institutions, and other organizations. For more information, please contact the Special Markets Department at the Perseus Books Group, 11 Cambridge Center, Cambridge, MA 02142, or call (800) 255-1514 or (617) 252-5298, or e-mail j.mccrary@perseusbooks.com.

Text design by Lisa Kreinbrink
Set in 11-point Sabon by the Perseus Books Group

First printing, January 2003
1   2   3   4   5   6   7   8   9   10—06   05   04   03

Contents

A Letter to the Expectant Fathers Who Read This Book

In this book, we have tried to help you understand what a woman goes through during pregnancy and how you can help her deal with the things that are happening to her. Pregnancy changes can be overwhelming, and they certainly are life changing. In some parts, we focus more on your partner because she is the one who is pregnant. But it isn't all about her because we know you are also an important part of the pregnancy.

In one respect, this is a book about how you can help her have the best pregnancy possible. But we have tried to include information on how pregnancy affects *you*, emotionally, physically and in other life-changing ways. We have provided many ideas and a great deal of information to help you through this time of change.

We hope we have achieved our goal of making pregnancy a more significant and understandable process for you, so you can share these 9 months in a meaningful way with the mother of your child.

Note to Readers

In this book, we have chosen not to discuss some of the more serious conditions and problems a woman may experience during a pregnancy. Most of them are dealt with in our other books, and you can read those for information on a particular situation.

The focus of this book is to provide you with vital information that is fairly elementary in nature to help you understand what may occur during a normal pregnancy, what you may need to be prepared for and how you can help your partner.

You're Expecting, Too, Dad!

You have probably recently learned that you're going to be a father. This may be exciting to you, or you may feel somewhat removed or on "the outside." There's no right or wrong way to feel—your emotions relate to your personal experiences. However, it is important to point out that you *are* part of this pregnancy. Although only the woman carries the baby, you, as her partner, can be a valuable asset to her throughout the months ahead.

In this book, we have attempted to explore pregnancy from your perspective—the male point of view. We provide you with information so you can be an informed participant and you can help make knowledgeable decisions regarding many aspects of pregnancy, labor and delivery. We give you ideas on ways to support your partner as she goes through the many changes that pregnancy brings. We supply you with hints and tips to help make your life, and hers, easier and more enjoyable. In short, we have tried to make the pregnancy experience a good one for you both.

Your partner is carrying *your* baby, so you are expecting, too! Help provide for your partner's and growing baby's well-being and safety. Bolster her spirits when she's feeling overwhelmed or down. Accept, with grace, the changes you may notice during her pregnancy—from mood swings to food cravings. Help her stay fit and healthy so she gives birth to a healthy baby. Support her in any way you can, without expecting too much in return. Remember—it's for the good of your baby!

An Explanation of Recurring Boxes

In each chapter, we have included recurring boxes. The titles are always the same, but the information changes. You will find two boxes that advise you what to do and what not to do—they are titled *Brownie Points* (things to do) and *In the Doghouse* (things not to do).

My Mother-in-Law Said boxes contain some debunked myths; you might hear them spoken by others. We jestingly titled it from your mother-in-law, but these words of *non*wisdom can be spoken by anyone who may not know what's really going on in a pregnancy (especially *yours!*).

The final boxes, *Memorable Moments from Dr. Dad*, are stories Dr. Curtis has gathered through his more than 20 years of guiding and assisting expectant couples through their pregnancies, as well as the births of his own five children. Some stories may cause you to laugh; others may bring a tear to your eye. Each reveals how differently pregnancy affects those who experience it.

The Big Picture

A Quick Look at Pregnancy, Birth and Beyond

1ST TRIMESTER—BEGINNING OF PREGNANCY THROUGH WEEK 13

The Good Part	*You May Have to Help Your Partner Deal With*	*Pay Attention To*
A positive pregnancy test, page 7	Emotional changes, page 52	Tests your partner may have, page 113
1st visit with the doctor, page 114	Fatigue, page 52	Nutrition, page 27
Telling family and friends	Morning sickness, page 58	Exercise, page 36
Hearing baby's heartbeat, page 115	Frequent urination, page 54	Safety issues, page 69
Great sex, page 96	Constipation, page 51	Smoking around your partner, pages 42, 43
Dreaming about the future together	Skin changes, page 61	Going to prenatal appointments, when possible, page 128
Partner's body begins to change and becomes more voluptuous, page 65	Helping your partner avoid smoking and alcohol use, pages 40, 43	Instructions and advice from the doctor
Growing closer from sharing the pregnancy experience	Changing the cat's litter box, page 69	Any medications your partner uses
Your partner's pregnancy "glow"	Avoiding saunas and hot tubs, page 70	Ways to help make life easier for your partner and yourself
Looking forward to, and making plans about, becoming a family	Cutting down on caffeine, page 34	
	Pregnancy problems, page 169	

2ND TRIMESTER—WEEKS 14 TO 26

The Good Part	*You May Have to Help Your Partner Deal With*	*Pay Attention To*
Your partner may feel great, and life may be very good	Her growing pregnancy and changing body, page 65	Prenatal visits and lab tests, page 114
Morning sickness is better, page 58	A new wardrobe	Exercising together, page 36
Feeling baby move for the first time, page 94	Lab tests results, page 114	Making things safe at home, page 69
Ultrasound of the baby, page 116	Changing emotions and mood swings, page 52	Helping your partner avoid falls, page 175
Your partner doesn't have periods and doesn't need contraception	Amniocentesis and other testing procedures, page 113	A good nutrition plan, page 28
This is a good time to travel because your partner will feel fairly well, page 80	Standing too long at any one time, pages 61, 68	Instructions and advice from the doctor
The pregnancy begins to show, and people will know your partner is pregnant	Swelling of her hands and feet, pages 62, 63	Signing up for childbirth-education classes, page 207
Picking baby names	Pregnancy problems, page 169	Checking into the daycare situation in your area, page 193
Sharing the ups and downs of pregnancy	Getting enough rest, page 52	Health insurance requirements and coverage, page 147
	Learning to sleep on her side	Learning about, and using, some good massage techniques, page 103

3ᴿᴰ TRIMESTER—WEEKS 27 TO 40

The Good Part	*You May Have to Help Your Partner Deal With*	*Pay Attention To*
Childbirth-education classes, page 207	Making plans to get to the hospital, page 220	Getting plenty of rest yourself
Tour of labor and delivery, page 209	More frequent appointments with the doctor	Plans for staying in touch with each other, page 217
Fixing up baby's nursery, page 197	False labor, page 221	Plans for getting to the hospital
Buying baby things, page 195	Visiting labor and delivery	How much time you will take off after delivery, page 83
Meeting the pediatrician, page 190	Hemorrhoids and other conditions, page 56	Getting a safe car seat and learning about its proper use, page 200
Dreaming about the future with your son	Emotional changes and mood swings, page 52	Preregistering at the hospital, page 220
Dreaming about the future with your daughter	Discomfort due to her increasing size	Instructions and advice from the doctor
The end of pregnancy is drawing near, and your baby will soon be born	New sexual positions, page 97	Practicing what you learn in childbirth-education classes, page 212
Making plans for baby's future	Pregnancy problems, page 169	
Deciding on baby's name	Finding daycare in advance, page 193	
	Not delivering by the due date	

LABOR AND DELIVERY

The Good Part	*You May Have to Help Your Partner Deal With*	*Pay Attention To*
Helping your partner deal with labor and delivery, page 214	Timing contractions, page 220	Packing *your* bag for the hospital, page 218
Cutting the umbilical cord, if you choose to do so, page 215	The pain of labor and delivery, page 223	Using massage techniques you have learned, page 224
Calling family and friends with news of baby's arrival, page 215	Deciding what type of pain relief she can use, if she chooses, page 223	Having a list of telephone numbers, enough change or a calling card to notify family and friends of baby's arrival
Seeing your baby	The length of labor	
Holding your baby	A Cesarean section, page 231	
Feeling your baby	Deciding whether to have a son circumcised, page 235	Your actions during labor—stay in labor and delivery; don't leave, page 214
Smelling your baby		
Baby's first pictures		
Relaxing with your partner	Physical changes after the birth	
Enjoying baby	Fatigue	
Showing your partner how proud of her you are	Taking care of baby	Remembering to bring your camera to take pictures, if you both agree on it, page 214
	Breastfeeding, page 237	
Sharing this wondrous experience	Being away from her job	
Falling in love with your baby		Bring your partner something special, such as flowers or a food treat

AT HOME WITH BABY

The Good Part	You May Have to Help Your Partner Deal With	Pay Attention To
Baby is finally home Beginning your life as a family Sex happens again, page 254 Bonding with your baby, page 242 Taking care of baby, page 247 Learning from your baby, page 252 Introducing baby to siblings Getting to know baby Adding the role of "dad" to your personal description	Baby blues or postpartum depression, page 257 Contraception, page 255 Lack of sleep, page 247 Accepting her new figure—it takes time to get back into shape Getting ready to go back to work Finding daycare Adjusting to life at home, if your partner doesn't work or doesn't return to work	Any excessive bleeding your partner experiences after she comes home Follow-up visits for mom and baby Always putting baby in the car seat when you travel in the car, page 200 Setting aside time for you and your partner, page 253 Asking for help if either you or your partner need it, page 242 Your own fatigue, page 247 Making your home safe, page 249 Being considerate of each other's feelings, page 251 How *your* role will change if *you* stay home Your feelings of depression, page 259

1

Essential Pregnancy Information

You're going to be a father!

You may be surprised.
You may be excited.
You may be nervous.

Chances are, you're somewhat bowled over by the mystery and uncertainties that lie ahead. That's OK—it's normal to feel many different emotions at this time.

Pregnancy is exciting and a little scary at the same time. It is a new, thrilling adventure for you and your partner, and it will be exciting for your family and friends, too. Make yourself an important part of this unique time. Read this book and our other books, try our suggestions, be a great expectant father, and soon you'll be an all-star dad!

Your pregnancy as a couple is exciting. It can also be a moving experience for you both. During these 9 months, together you'll watch the growth of your baby as your partner grows bigger.

Big changes are on the way. You may not realize it yet, but your life will soon change forever. How you define yourself professionally

---

Chapter Focus

In this chapter, we provide you with tools you need to become informed about pregnancy. This is a time of great change in your partner, most of which you'll be able to see. It's also a time of incredible growth and development of the fetus, which you won't be able to see, except through various tests.

By being informed about what pregnancy actually is, the various physical changes your partner may experience, tests she might have and the importance of attending office visits, you'll have a better understanding of what's happening. We also have compiled *20 Top Tips for Expectant Dads*, which is a list of things you can do together to make this pregnancy a great one for everyone!

This chapter provides you with some basic information about pregnancy so you can be knowledgeable about what will occur in the months ahead.

and personally will change to add the role of "father-to-be." Soon, you'll be "dad." Being a father is one of the most wonderful and important jobs you'll ever have.

WHAT IS PREGNANCY?

You probably have a pretty good idea of what pregnancy is—the condition in which a woman carries a developing fetus in her womb (uterus) for about 266 days, until the baby is developed and ready to be born. But as you'll learn during these next months, pregnancy involves a lot of areas you might not have considered. Your partner's health impacts greatly on her pregnancy experience and the health of your growing baby; you may be asked to participate in exercise programs or special meal plans to help her in her efforts. She'll need your support in many other areas, too, so be prepared for requests that may be made of you. Anything you do to help your pregnant partner during this time also helps your growing baby! Work on this together.

> **Find the Definition**
>
> As you read this book, if you come across a term you are unfamiliar with, or want to know the definition of, see the section *Pregnancy-Related Terms for Expecting Couples* that begins on page 15. Although this first chapter is fairly basic and easy to understand, we do use some terms you may need to check out. Refer to this section as you read through the book, if you find other terms you need clarified.

As you and your partner progress through your pregnancy as a couple, you'll probably hear and read lots of words and terms you're unfamiliar with. You may come across them in our other books, at prenatal visits and in childbirth-education classes. Women who have not been pregnant before (or even experienced moms) may be as confused about some of the definitions as you might be. We have defined many terms you may hear during these next months. Knowing what they mean can give you a sense of security (and superiority) when it comes to discussing various pregnancy issues. Learn these things together when you can. Who knows—you may end up knowing more about what's going on during pregnancy and you'll be explaining things to your pregnant partner! See the collection of *Pregnancy-Related Terms for Expecting Couples* that begins on page 15.

YOUR BABY'S DUE DATE

One term you'll probably become familiar with during your pregnancy is the *due date*. This is the anticipated date your child will probably be born. We say "anticipated date" because only 5% of all babies are actually born on the due date. Determining the due date is not an exact science; there are a lot of factors that come into play during pregnancy that can affect the date.

However, estimating the due date is important for a few reasons. First, it provides an expected date for baby's arrival, which can help prepare you mentally and emotionally for the birth of your baby. Second, it helps estimate baby's growth; it may indicate when a baby is overdue or when a woman goes into premature labor. Third, it serves as a marker for your doctor to help determine when to perform certain tests or procedures.

Determining the Due Date

Most couples don't know the exact date their baby was conceived, but the woman often knows the day her last menstrual period began. The doctor adds 2 weeks to the first day of the last period as an estimate of when conception occurred. The estimated due date is 38 weeks after the date of conception (40 weeks after the first day of the woman's last period).

You can also figure the due date by adding 7 days to the date your partner's last menstrual period began, then subtracting 3 months. This gives you the approximate date of delivery. For example, if her last period began on January 20, her estimated due date is October 27.

The best way to think about a due date is that it is a goal you are working toward. You can make plans about the pregnancy, prepare for labor and delivery, work out the details of financial changes and get ready for your baby's arrival. When baby arrives, you'll be ready!

A WOMAN GOES THROUGH MANY CHANGES DURING PREGNANCY

Your pregnant partner will experience a lot of changes in the months ahead; this is a normal part of the pregnancy process. By knowing about expected changes, you may be more comfortable with them, and you can also be more helpful and supportive.

In the first part of pregnancy, you won't see many physical changes. However, as a couple, you may feel a new freedom in your relationship. There's no need for birth control now that you are pregnant. For many couples, this time can be very romantic. You may also see the pregnancy as an accomplishment—you may have been concerned about getting pregnant together, but now you've done it! You may feel that pregnancy is a statement of your manhood as much as it is of your partner's womanhood.

BROWNIE POINTS

It's important to be sympathetic when your partner suffers from some of the common discomforts of pregnancy, including morning sickness, fatigue, sore breasts or having to go to the bathroom all the time. These are *not* in her head—they are real conditions. Your understanding can help make her feel a lot better!

By the beginning of the 4th month, people will be able to tell your partner is pregnant. One of the most exciting things in pregnancy happens around this time. Your partner begins to feel your baby move! This can be a very exciting and emotional time for you both. (You may be able to feel baby's movements later in pregnancy by placing your hands on your partner's abdomen when baby is active. That can be exciting for you, too.)

During the latter part of pregnancy, you'll see many changes. Your baby will be growing quite a bit and gaining a great deal of weight, in preparation for birth. This growth can cause discomfort for the pregnant woman, so it's a time to be sympathetic, helpful and supportive. It's not "all in her head."

By being aware of various changes that occur during pregnancy, you can help your partner cope with many of them. It can help you be more understanding about why she is crying sometimes, doesn't feel well enough to make dinner at other times or just can't go anywhere until she takes a nap. One thing will soon become evident—when one member of the team is unhappy, the entire team is unhappy.

Be patient when unusual situations arise. Your partner is going through a lot right now. The hormones that her body releases to support the pregnancy can affect her in many different ways! They're not an excuse; they're an explanation. See our complete

> ### My Mother-in-Law Said
>
> *If a pregnant woman reaches over her head, the umbilical cord may get wrapped around the baby's neck.*
>
> The truth is that there is nothing a pregnant woman can do to cause this problem, and there's nothing she can do to prevent it.

discussion in Chapter 3 of physical changes and common discomforts that can occur during pregnancy, and learn about ways you and your partner can deal with them.

TESTS FOR YOUR PREGNANCY

The Pregnancy Test

The first test you and your partner may take is a home pregnancy test. A pregnancy test can be positive (show a woman is pregnant) even before a woman misses her menstrual period. Today, some home pregnancy tests are so effective that they can provide a 99% accurate test result *3 days before* a menstrual period is expected! However, we recommend you wait until your partner misses her period before taking a test to save both of you emotional energy and some money.

When your pregnancy test is positive, celebrate! A positive pregnancy test is a time to be excited. Your reaction may tell your partner a lot about how you feel about being pregnant together. Some women are shocked and a little scared when their pregnancy test is positive. Their first thought is, "What do we do now?" Be smart and answer, "Call the doctor for an appointment."

Routine Pregnancy Tests Done by the Doctor

Your pregnancy doctor will probably order several tests at your partner's first prenatal visit. We cover all the pregnancy tests in depth in Chapter 6; you can also find them defined in the section *Pregnancy-Related Terms for Expecting Couples* that begins on page 15. Some routine tests ordered for nearly every woman during her first pregnancy include a complete blood count (CBC), urinalysis and urine culture, blood typing, a test for syphilis, cervical cultures, rubella titers, Rh-factor, a test for hepatitis-B antibodies, a Pap smear and ultrasound.

IN THE DOGHOUSE

During pregnancy, a woman is *supposed* to gain weight—a normal-weight woman should gain between 25 and 35 pounds. Don't comment on your partner's weight, food intake or exercise routine. Be helpful and encouraging, but don't hassle her or make jokes about how much weight she gains.

If your partner has been pregnant before, some of the tests, such as for Rh-factor, a blood type or a rubella titer, probably will not be done again. Other tests are done every time she goes to the office for a prenatal visit, including a blood-pressure check, a urine check and a weight check.

The tests listed above are usually done in the office or a lab and may not require your presence, unless you believe your partner may need your support. An exception is the ultrasound test; most couples want to share this together.

Other Tests May Be Ordered

Today, we have many specialized tests to use during pregnancy to check a woman's health and the health of her growing baby. These special tests can range from a simple test done on a woman's blood to more invasive tests, in which amniotic fluid or tissue is taken from the uterus through the abdomen or vagina.

As a couple, you may want to discuss some tests with your pregnancy doctor. These tests are more specialized and are ordered when they are indicated. These tests are covered in more depth in Chapter 6; you can also find them defined in the section *Pregnancy-Related Terms for Expecting Couples* that begins on page 15. Some of the more specialized tests include amniocentesis, chorionic villus sampling, alpha-fetoprotein test (AFP), blood-sugar tests, triple-screen test, quad-screen test, fetal fibronectin (fFN) test, fetoscopy, nonstress test, contraction-stress test, biophysical profile and others.

A few of these tests can be very stressful for a pregnant couple, especially the woman. If your partner must undergo some of the more invasive tests, plan to be with her for them. In some cases, she will need your emotional support. In others, she may be temporarily physically disabled and will need you to take her home and to care for her.

Ask your pregnancy doctor which tests he or she would advise you to attend. Let the doctor know you would like to discuss test results at a prenatal visit, so you and your partner have a clear understanding of why each test was done and what results show.

AN OVERVIEW OF PREGNANCY AND SOME OF THE PEOPLE INVOLVED

Prenatal care is the care a woman receives during pregnancy. *Prenatal* means *before birth*. This special care is necessary to help discover any pregnancy problems and to address them before they become serious. As a couple, you and your partner want to feel confident that the care is the best you can find; then you'll both be able to relax and enjoy your pregnancy. It really is a special time in your life and an enjoyable one, too. You also want to do everything possible to make it the best time for your growing baby.

Choosing a Healthcare Provider

There are many choices when it comes to choosing a healthcare provider for pregnancy. Choices include an obstetrician, a family practitioner or a certified nurse-midwife to oversee prenatal care. In special high-risk pregnancies, a woman may need to see a perinatologist.

An *obstetrician* (often referred to as an *OB/GYN*) is a medical doctor or osteopathic physician who specializes in the care of pregnant women, including delivering babies. He or she has completed further training in obstetrics and gynecology after medical school.

> ## Your Pregnancy Doctor
>
> Although the doctor you and your partner choose as your pregnancy doctor probably isn't someone you would see for medical problems, think of this professional as taking care of the growing baby, your partner and you! You're part of this pregnancy, so don't hesitate to ask questions or to seek advice from the doctor or his or her office staff about things that concern you. It's important for you to feel comfortable with this person, too.

A *family practitioner,* sometimes called a *general practitioner,* often provides care for the entire family. Many family practitioners deliver babies and are very experienced. In some cases, an obstetrician may not be available in a community because it is small or remote so a family practitioner often delivers babies. If problems arise, a family practitioner may refer a pregnant woman to an obstetrician for prenatal care.

A *certified nurse-midwife* is a trained nursing professional who cares for women who have low-risk, uncomplicated pregnancies and delivers their babies. These professionals are registered nurses who have received additional professional training and certification in nurse-midwifery. They are supervised by a physician and call him or her if complications occur.

A *perinatologist* is an obstetrician who specializes in high-risk pregnancies. Only about 10% of all pregnant women need to see one. If a serious pregnancy problem develops, a woman may be referred to a perinatologist.

A person who supports a woman during her labor and may act as her labor coach is called a *doula*. Most doulas are women who have previously given birth, so they are aware of many of the situations that can arise during childbirth. We discuss doulas in more depth in Chapter 9.

Attending Prenatal Visits

Your pregnancy doctor is specially trained to deal with pregnancy, labor and delivery. He or she can answer questions and deal with your concerns during this important time. Even though you are not the primary patient in this pregnancy, your partner's doctor should be willing to discuss *your* particular concerns and to answer *your* questions. That is why it's important for you to attend prenatal visits when you can. It gives you the opportunity to show your partner you support her, and you can seek answers to pregnancy issues that you may personally have. You may also want to read the in-depth discussion of office visits in Chapter 6.

MEMORABLE MOMENTS FROM DR. DAD

Steve and Natalie came to the office for an infertility consult. They were downcast because they had been trying for over 2 years to get pregnant, without results. Natalie commented that her breasts were a little sore, and she didn't feel quite right. She was wondering if her malaise could be caused by the fertility tests she had been undergoing. Her periods had always been irregular, and she mentioned it had been 2 months since her last period. Something told me we should do a pregnancy test, so we did one right there in the office. It was positive! With them both crying, we did a new pregnancy visit instead of an infertility consult! They left the office with prenatal vitamins instead of fertility drugs.

20 TOP TIPS FOR EXPECTANT DADS (FROM THOSE WHO'VE BEEN THERE)

1. Be a part of the pregnancy, right from the beginning. It helps you feel involved in what's going on, and it helps your partner realize you take this pregnancy seriously and want to help.

2. Learn about pregnancy, labor and delivery. Read this book and our other books, attend prenatal appointments and go to childbirth-education classes. That way you'll have a better understanding of what's going on, and you'll be able to be more supportive of your partner. And it'll be easier for you to ask questions or to express your concerns if you have information.

3. Be a good listener. Give your partner your undivided attention, and listen to her when she talks to you. Sometimes she may just want to talk about a situation or a problem. Sometimes she needs to vent. Sometimes she needs your reassurance. Be there for her.

4. Let your partner know how she can help *you!* You need encouragement, support and help, too. It's important to tell her what you need, when you need it.

5. Ask questions, and get answers. If either of you is concerned about something, don't let it nag at you. Find out what you want to know. If your question is not answered to your satisfaction by the doctor or the doctor's staff, keep asking it until you have an answer you can understand. Read our other pregnancy books, magazine articles and other informative material.

6. Don't tell your partner to stop worrying or try to keep her from expressing her emotions. Both go along with being pregnant. Instead, try to offer your support and to listen to her.

7. Be patient with your partner—she's going through a lot of changes right now. Your patience and understanding can go a long way in helping her deal with the changes she experiences.

8. Ask your partner to be patient with you—this is a new experience that may create situations you are unfamiliar with. You'll appreciate her patience when you attempt new things.

9. Tell your partner her pregnant body is beautiful. She has new curves and a softness you may not have seen before. Her changing body reflects the changes going on inside her. Don't tell her she looks big or make comments about her weight gain.

10. If *you* experience any pregnancy symptoms, called *couvade* (see page 77), don't fret about it. It's not unusual. Let your partner know what's going on—you'll be able to empathize with each other.

11. Try to keep stress in your lives to a minimum. Practice stress-relieving activities and exercises together. They can help you, too.

12. Make an attempt to keep romance alive. Go out to lunch or dinner together. Take a leisurely walk in the evening. Go to a movie or play. Keep it up after baby's birth.

13. When necessary, make changes in your lifestyle to support your partner. Give up smoking. Get lots of exercise. Eat nutritiously. When you work together, it helps both of you make healthy changes.

14. Don't take on new projects, add responsibilities to your plate or participate in activities that keep you apart a lot. Be as available as possible to share the pregnancy experience together.

15. Reassure your partner when she needs it. She may be concerned that something she did before pregnancy could harm the baby. She may feel she's not doing enough during the pregnancy to ensure a

BROWNIE POINTS

Supporting your partner through the months of pregnancy is one of the best gifts you can give your child. Take time to listen, help out and provide emotional support when you can. A healthy mom usually gives birth to a healthy baby.

healthy baby. She may worry that she won't be a good mother. These are all common concerns, so don't scoff at her anxiety. Sympathize with her, and let her know you are there to listen.

16. Tell your partner when you need some reassurance. You may feel unnerved by events that are occurring. If you're honest about your fears and uncertainties, you can work together to find solutions, and you'll both feel better.

17. Consider taking time off after baby's birth (paternity leave is covered in depth beginning on page 83). You can help out with baby while your partner recovers, or you may decide to stay at home with baby by yourself for a time after mom returns to work.

18. Learn about parenting. Read books, watch videos and talk with other dads. Although a woman may often be more involved with an infant, there's no reason you can't be just as involved and assume some of the parenting responsibilities after baby is born.

19. Don't try to be perfect. Pregnancy is probably a new experience for you, so allow yourself to learn as you go. You may make some mistakes, but everyone does, so relax.

20. Enjoy this pregnancy together. Once baby arrives, you'll have many demands on your time and attention. Use this wonderful time to grow closer as a couple.

Pregnancy-Related Terms for Expecting Couples

In this section, we have gathered together a lot of terms you and your partner may hear during pregnancy. Some of the terms pertain to pregnancy; some cover various tests a pregnant woman might have. Some relate to labor and delivery. A few terms apply to the time after baby's birth. We've divided terms into *Basic Pregnancy Information, Tests on Mother-to-Be and Baby, Labor and Delivery* and *After Baby's Birth*.

BASIC PREGNANCY INFORMATION

Amniotic fluid—Fluid surrounding the baby inside the amniotic sac.

Amniotic sac—Membrane that surrounds the baby inside the uterus. It contains the baby, placenta and amniotic fluid.

Areola—Pigmented or colored ring surrounding the nipple of the breast.

Blood pressure—Push of the blood against the walls of the arteries, which carry blood away from the heart. Changes in blood pressure may indicate problems.

Board certification (of physician)—Doctor has received additional training and testing in a particular specialty. In the area of obstetrics, the American College of Obstetricians and Gynecologists offers this training. Certification requires expertise in care of women. *FACOG* following a doctor's name means he or she is a Fellow of the American College of Obstetricians and Gynecologists.

Braxton-Hicks contractions—Irregular tightening of uterus during pregnancy.

Cervix—Opening of the uterus.

Chadwick's sign—Dark-blue or purple discoloration of the mucosa of the vagina and cervix during pregnancy.

Chloasma—Increased pigmentation or extensive brown patches of irregular shape and size on the face (commonly has the appearance of a butterfly) or other parts of the body. Also called *mask of pregnancy.*

Chromosomal abnormality—Abnormal number or abnormal makeup of chromosomes.

Chromosome—Thread in a cell's nucleus that contains DNA, which transmits genetic information.

Congenital problem—Problem present at birth.

Constipation—Infrequent or incomplete bowel movements.

Dilatation and curettage (D&C)—Surgical procedure in which the cervix is opened and tissue is scraped or suctioned out of the uterus.

Down syndrome—Chromosomal disorder in which the baby has three copies of Chromosome 21 (instead of two); results in mental retardation, distinct physical traits and various other problems.

Due date—Date baby is expected to be born. Most babies are born near this date, but only 1 of 20 are born on the actual date.

Eclampsia—Convulsions and coma in a woman with pre-eclampsia. See *pre-eclampsia.* Not related to epilepsy.

Ectopic pregnancy—Pregnancy that occurs outside the uterine cavity, most often in a Fallopian tube.

Embryo—Organism in the early stages of development; in a human pregnancy from conception to 10 weeks.

Embryonic period—First 10 weeks of gestation.

Fallopian tube—Tube that leads from the cavity of the uterus to the area of the ovary.

Fetal anomaly—Fetal malformation or abnormal development.

Fetal distress—Problems with the baby that occur before birth or during labor; often requires immediate delivery.

Fetal period—Time period following embryonic period (first 10 weeks of gestation) until birth.

Fetus—Unborn baby after 10 weeks of gestation until birth.

Fundus—Top part of the uterus; often measured during pregnancy.

Genes—Basic units of heredity. Each gene carries specific information and is passed from parent to child. A child receives half of its genes from its mother and half from its father. Every human has about 100,000 genes.

Genetic counseling—Consultation between a couple and specialists about genetic defects and the possibility of presence or recurrence of genetic problems in a pregnancy.

Gestational diabetes—Occurrence of diabetes during pregnancy (gestation).

Group-B streptococcal infection (GBS)—Infection occurring in the mother's vagina, throat or rectum. (Infection can be in any of these areas.) GBS can be serious for the baby.

Heartburn—Discomfort or pain that occurs in the chest, often after eating.

Hemorrhoids—Dilated blood vessels, most often found in or around the rectum.

High-risk pregnancy—Pregnancy with complications that require individualized medical attention, often from a specialist. See *perinatologist.*

Human chorionic gonadotropin—Hormone produced in early pregnancy that is measured by a pregnancy test or quantitative HCG test.

Hyperemesis gravidarum—Severe nausea, dehydration and vomiting during pregnancy. Occurs most frequently during the first trimester.

Hypertension, pregnancy-induced—High blood pressure that occurs during pregnancy.

Intrauterine-growth restriction (IUGR)—Inadequate growth of the fetus during pregnancy. Previously called *intrauterine-growth retardation.*

Iron-deficiency anemia—Anemia produced by lack of iron in the diet; often seen in pregnancy.

Isoimmunization—Development of specific antibodies directed at the red blood cells of another individual, such as a baby in the uterus. Occurs when an Rh-negative woman carries an Rh-positive baby or when she is given Rh-positive blood.

Lightening—Change in the shape of the pregnant uterus a few weeks before labor. Often described as the baby "dropping."

Linea nigra—Line of increased pigmentation that often develops during pregnancy; line runs down the abdomen from bellybutton to pubic area.

Miscarriage—Termination or premature end of pregnancy. Giving birth to an embryo or fetus before it can live outside the womb, usually defined as before 20 weeks of pregnancy.

Morning sickness—Nausea and vomiting, primarily during the first trimester of pregnancy. See also *hyperemesis gravidarum.*

Neural-tube defects—Abnormalities in development of the fetal spinal cord and brain.

Nurse–midwife—Registered nurse who has received extra training in the care of pregnant women and the delivery of babies.

Obstetrician—Physician who specializes in the care of pregnant women and the delivery of babies.

Perinatologist—Physician who specializes in the care of high-risk pregnancies.

Placenta—Organ that develops inside the uterus during pregnancy that is attached to the baby by the umbilical cord. Essential for the baby's growth and development.

Placenta previa—Low attachment of the placenta, covering all or part of the cervix.

Placental abruption—Premature separation of the placenta from the uterus.

Postdate birth—Baby born 2 weeks or more past its due date.

Pre-eclampsia—Combination of symptoms unique to pregnancy, including high blood pressure, edema, swelling and changes in reflexes.

Premature delivery—Delivery before 38 weeks gestation.

Prenatal care—Program of care for a pregnant woman before the birth of her baby.

Pubic symphysis—Bony prominence in the pelvic bone found in the middle of a woman's lower abdomen. Landmark from which the doctor often measures the growing uterus during pregnancy.

Quickening—Mother-to-be's feeling the baby move inside her uterus.

Rh-negative—Absence of rhesus antibody in the blood.

Rho-GAM—Medication given during pregnancy and following delivery to prevent isoimmunization. See *isoimmunization*.

Round-ligament pain—Pain caused by ligament on the sides of the uterus stretching during pregnancy.

Stillbirth—Death of a fetus before birth, usually defined as after 20 weeks gestation.

Stretch marks—Areas of the skin that are stretched during pregnancy. Often found on the abdomen, breasts, buttocks and legs.

Term—Baby is considered "term" when it is born after 38 weeks. Also called *full term*.

Trimester—Three-month period of time. Pregnancy is divided into three equal periods (trimesters) of about 13 weeks each.

Umbilical cord—Cord that connects the placenta to the developing baby. It removes waste products and carbon dioxide from the baby and brings oxygenated blood and nutrients from the mother through the placenta to the baby.

Uterus—Organ an embryo/fetus grows in. Also called a *womb*.

Vagina—Birth canal.

Varicose veins—Blood vessels (veins) that are dilated or enlarged.

Vena cava—Major vein in the body that empties into the right atrium of the heart. It returns unoxygenated blood to the heart for transport to the lungs.

TESTS ON MOTHER-TO-BE AND BABY

Abdominal measurement—Measurement taken of the growth of the baby in the uterus at prenatal visits. Measurement is from the pubic symphysis to the fundus. Too much growth or too little growth may indicate problems.

Alpha-fetoprotein (AFP)—Substance produced by the unborn baby as it grows inside the uterus; found in maternal blood and amniotic fluid. Larger-than-normal amounts are found in mother's blood if fetus has neural-tube defects.

Amniocentesis—Process by which amniotic fluid is removed from the amniotic sac for testing. Fluid is tested for some genetic defects and for fetal lung maturity.

Biophysical profile—Method of evaluating a fetus before birth.

Blood typing—Test to determine if a woman's blood type is A, B, AB or O.

Blood-pressure check—High blood pressure can be significant during pregnancy, especially nearer the due date. Changes in blood-pressure readings can alert the doctor to potential problems.

Blood-sugar tests—See *glucose-tolerance test.*

Canavan's disease screening—Blood test performed on people of Ashkenazi Jewish background to determine if a fetus is affected with Canavan's disease.

Cervical cultures—To test for STDs; when a Pap smear is done, a sample may also be taken to check for chlamydia, gonorrhea or other STDs.

Chorionic villus sampling (CVS)—Diagnostic test that can be done early in pregnancy to determine pregnancy abnormalities. A biopsy of tissue is taken from inside the uterus through the abdomen or the cervix.

Complete blood count (CBC)—Blood test to check the mother's iron stores and for infections.

Congenital deafness screening—If a couple has a family history of inherited deafness, this blood test may identify the problem before baby's birth.

Contraction-stress test—Response of fetus to uterine contractions; used to evaluate fetal well-being.

Doppler—Device that enhances the fetal heartbeat so the doctor and others can hear it.

Familial Mediterranean fever screening—Blood test performed on people of Armenian, Arabic, Turkish and Sephardic Jewish background to identify carriers of the recessive gene. Permits diagnosis in a newborn so treatment can be started.

Fetal fibronectin (fFN)—Test done to evaluate premature labor. A sample of cervical-vaginal secretions is taken; if fFN is present after 22 weeks, it indicates increased risk for preterm delivery.

Fetal monitor—Device used before or during labor to listen to and record the fetal heartbeat. Monitoring baby inside the uterus can be *external* (through maternal abdomen) or *internal* (through maternal vagina).

Fetoscopy—Test that enables doctor to look through a fetoscope (a fiber-optics scope) to detect subtle abnormalities and problems in a fetus while it is still inside the mother's uterus.

Genetics tests—Various screening and diagnostic tests done to determine whether a couple might have a child with a genetic defect. Usually part of genetic counseling.

Glucose-tolerance test—Done to evaluate a body's response to sugar. Blood is drawn from the mother-to-be once or at intervals following ingestion of a sugary substance.

Group-B streptococcus (GBS) test—Near the end of pregnancy, samples may be taken from the expectant woman's vagina, perineum and rectum to check for GBS. A urine test may also be done. If the test is positive, treatment may be started or given during labor.

Hepatitis-B antibodies test—Determines if the pregnant woman has ever been exposed to hepatitis-B.

HIV/AIDS test—To determine if a woman has HIV or AIDS (the test cannot be done without the woman's knowledge *and* permission).

Home uterine monitoring—Contractions of a pregnant woman's uterus are recorded at home, then transmitted by telephone to the doctor (no special equipment is needed). Used to identify women at risk of premature labor.

Imaging tests—Tests that look inside the body, including ultrasound, X-rays, CT scans or CAT scans, and magnetic resonance imaging (MRI).

Kick count—Record of how often a pregnant woman feels her baby move; used to evaluate fetal well-being.

Multiple-markers test—See *quad-screen test* and *triple-screen test*.

Nonstress test—Test in which movements of the baby felt by the mother or observed by a healthcare provider are recorded, along with changes in the fetal heart rate. Used to evaluate fetal well-being.

Nuchal translucency screening—Detailed ultrasound that allows the doctor to measure the space behind baby's neck. Combined with blood test results, it can measure a woman's risk of having a baby with Down syndrome.

Pap smear—Early screening test for cervical cancer.

Pelvic exam—Physical examination by the doctor who feels inside a woman's pelvic area. Used to evaluate the size of the uterus at the beginning of pregnancy and to help the doctor determine if the cervix is dilating and thinning toward the end of pregnancy.

Percutaneous umbilical blood sampling (cordocentesis)—Test done on the fetus to diagnose Rh-incompatibility, blood disorders and infections.

Quad-screen test—Measurement of four blood components to help identify problems. The four tests include alpha-fetoprotein, human chorionic gonadotropin, unconjugated estriol and inhibin-A, a chemical produced by the ovaries and placenta.

Rh-factor—Blood test to determine if a woman is Rh-negative.

Rubella titers—Blood test to check for immunity against rubella (German measles).

Sonogram or sonography—See *ultrasound*.

Stress test—Test in which mild contractions of the mother's uterus are induced; fetal heart rate in response to the contractions is noted. Also called *contraction-stress test* or *CST*.

Syphilis test—To test for syphilis; if a woman has syphilis, treatment will be started.

Triple-screen test—Measurement of three blood components to help identify problems. The three tests include alpha-fetoprotein, human chorionic gonadotropin and unconjugated estriol, a form of estrogen produced by the placenta.

Ultrasound—Noninvasive test that shows a picture of fetus inside womb. Sound waves bounce off fetus to create a picture.

Urinalysis and urine cultures—To test for any infections and to determine the levels of sugar and protein in the urine.

Weight check—Weight is checked at every prenatal visit; gaining too much weight or not gaining enough weight can indicate problems.

LABOR AND DELIVERY

Active labor—When a woman is dilated between 4 and 8cm. Contractions are usually 3 to 5 minutes apart.

Afterbirth—Placenta and membranes expelled after baby is delivered. See *placenta.*

Augmented labor—When labor is "stalled" or progress is not being made during labor, medication (oxytocin) is given.

Back labor—Pain of labor felt in lower back.

Birthing center—Facility specializing in the delivery of babies. Usually a woman labors, delivers and recovers in the same room. It may be part of a hospital or a freestanding unit. Sometimes called LDRP, for *labor, delivery, recovery* and *postpartum.*

Bishop score—Method used to predict the success of inducing labor. Includes dilatation, effacement, station, consistency and position of the cervix. A score is given for each point, and they are added together to give a total score to help doctor decide whether to induce labor.

Bloody show—Small amount of vaginal bleeding late in pregnancy; often precedes labor.

Breech presentation—Abnormal birth position of the fetus. Buttocks or legs come into the birth canal before the head.

Cesarean section or delivery—Delivery of a baby through an abdominal incision rather than through the vagina.

Contractions—Uterus squeezes or tightens to push the baby out of the uterus during birth.

Dilatation—How much the cervix has opened before the birth. When a woman is fully dilated, she is at 10cm.

Early labor—When a woman experiences regular contractions (one every 20 minutes increasing to one every 5 minutes) for longer than 2 hours. The cervix usually dilates to 3 or 4cm.

Effacement—Thinning of cervix; occurs during labor.

Enema—Fluid injected into the rectum to clear the bowel.

Epidural block—Type of anesthesia inserted into the area around the spinal cord during labor.

Episiotomy—Surgical incision of the perineum (area between the vagina and the rectum). Used during delivery to avoid tearing vaginal opening and rectum.

External cephalic version (ECV)—Procedure done late in pregnancy, in which doctor manually attempts to move a baby in the breech presentation into the normal head-down birth position.

False labor—Tightening of uterus without dilatation of the cervix.

Forceps—Instrument sometimes used to deliver baby. It is placed around the baby's head, inside the birth canal, to help guide the baby out of the birth canal during delivery.

Induced labor—Labor started using a medication. See *oxytocin*.

Labor—Process of expelling fetus from the uterus.

Lochia—Vaginal discharge that occurs after delivery of the baby and placenta.

Mucus plug—Secretions in the cervix; often released just before labor.

Natural childbirth—Labor and delivery in which mother remains awake to help deliver her baby. Some people believe that with natural childbirth, a woman cannot ask for pain-relief medication; however, this is untrue. The woman may have taken classes to prepare her for labor and delivery.

Oxytocin—Medication that causes uterine contractions; used to induce or augment labor. It may be called by its brand name *Pitocin*. Also the hormone produced by pituitary glands.

Paracervical block—Local anesthetic to relieve pain of cervical dilatation.

Perineum—Area between the rectum and vagina.

Prepared childbirth—Woman has taken classes so she knows what to expect during labor and delivery. She may request pain medication if she needs it.

Presentation—Describes which part of the baby comes into the birth canal first.

Pudendal block—Local anesthesia during labor.

Rupture of membranes—Loss of fluid from the amniotic sac. Also called *breaking of waters* or *water breaking.*

Silent labor—Painless dilatation of the cervix.

Station—Estimation of the baby's descent in the birth canal in preparation for birth.

Transition—Phase after active labor during which the cervix fully dilates. Contractions are strongest during this stage.

Vacuum extractor—Device sometimes used to provide traction on fetal head during delivery; used to help deliver a baby.

AFTER BABY'S BIRTH

Apgar scores—Measurement of a baby's response to birth and life on its own. Taken 1 minute and 5 minutes after birth.

Bilirubin—Yellow or orange pigment in bile.

Baby blues—Mild depression in woman after delivery.

Colostrum—Thin, yellow fluid first produced by the breasts. Most often seen toward the end of pregnancy. It is different in content from milk produced later during nursing.

Engorgement—Filled with fluid; usually refers to breast engorgement in a breastfeeding mother.

Expressing breast milk—Manually forcing milk out of the breast.

Jaundice—Yellow staining of the skin, sclera (eyes) and deeper tissues of the body. Caused by excessive amounts of bilirubin.

Meconium—First intestinal discharge of the newborn; dark green or yellow in color. It consists of epithelial or surface cells, mucus and bile. Discharge may occur before or during labor or soon after birth.

Pediatrician—Physician who specializes in the care of babies and children.

Postpartum—The 6-week period following a baby's birth. Refers to the mother, not the baby.

Postpartum distress syndrome—Range of symptoms including baby blues, postpartum depression and postpartum psychosis.

2

Lifestyle Changes for You as an Expecting Couple

Now that your pregnancy is becoming a reality, it's time to analyze the situation to find ways to help you and your partner have a happy, healthy pregnancy. You want a healthy baby. That's the goal in every pregnancy—a healthy mom and a healthy baby.

Ways to help ensure that your baby is healthy revolve around the good health of the mother-to-be. This includes her nutrition plan, her exercise program, her environment and her emotional well-being. As an expectant dad, you can be a very important part of each activity. You can promote good nutrition, participate with her in some form of exercise, keep your environment and hers healthy and safe, and support her emotionally.

Many couples have said that some of their fondest memories from pregnancy come from adjustments they had to make in their lifestyles. Some of these changes could become part of your life together, even after your baby is born.

Chapter Focus

In this chapter, we provide you with tips on eating healthfully together and ideas for exercising as a couple. We also suggest some lifestyle changes that may need to be made and give you insights on ways to support your partner. We hope these ideas will help make her life, and yours, pleasant and hassle-free while helping to ensure a happy, healthy pregnancy.

A HEALTHY NUTRITION PLAN IS ESSENTIAL

Good maternal nutrition is one of the most important keys to a healthy baby. When a mom-to-be eats wisely and nutritiously, her growing fetus receives the nutrients it needs to develop and grow into a healthy baby. You can be a part of this process by encouraging your partner to eat healthfully.

Have you heard the saying, "A pregnant woman is eating for two"? It's true, she is eating for two—herself and her baby—but she doesn't have to eat *twice* as much! Some people have this misconception, but the truth is if a woman is average weight when she begins her pregnancy, she only needs to eat about 300 additional calories a day to provide good nutrition for her baby. That's not a lot of food—a woman can add those extra 300 calories by eating one 8-ounce carton of low-fat yogurt and a medium apple.

Help your partner by eating healthy foods yourself. Don't ask her to make high-calorie foods for you and expect her to eat a different menu. Don't suggest that you both catch a quick meal by stopping at a fast-food restaurant on a regular basis. Make the commitment now to eat healthy foods that will benefit all of you.

What Foods Should We Eat?

A variety of foods in your daily diet will supply the nutrients needed for a healthy pregnancy. A healthful nutrition plan includes dairy products, protein foods, fruits and vegetables, and breads and cereals. It may take some planning, but together you can develop a meal plan that is beneficial for you both. A healthy eating plan can also help you watch your weight or avoid high-calorie, non-nutritious foods.

Below is a list of daily servings from six food groups. Together, use the list to help you develop a good nutrition plan and to prepare a diverse menu:

✓ dairy products—4 to 5 servings a day

✓ protein sources—3 to 4 servings a day (6 to 7 ounces; 168 to 196g)

✓ vegetables—at least 4 servings a day

✓ fruits—2 to 4 servings a day

✓ breads, cereal, pasta and rice—6 to 11 servings a day

✓ fats/flavorings—3 to 5 servings a day

You might want to sit down together and make a meal plan for the week. Consider the foods above and the number of servings required, and decide what foods and recipes will fill these needs. Although this may not be something you have done together in the past, making and carrying out this plan together can help strengthen your relationship. It shows your partner you care about her health and your growing baby's health, and you are working together toward the important goal of eating well.

How Much Calcium?

It may be a little difficult for your partner to determine how much calcium she is getting from the foods she eats. Package labeling usually lists the *percentage* of calcium contained in a food. This may be confusing because it's hard to know how much that is.

The solution is to understand that labeling is based on the RDA's recommendation for a nonpregnant woman, which is 800mg a day. If a package states "calcium 20%," just multiply 800 times 0.2, which gives you the amount of 160mg. Your partner can keep a written record of how much calcium she receives from each calcium-containing food she eats. A pregnant woman needs a total of about 1200mg of calcium a day.

Some Good Food Choices

TO BUILD BABY'S BRAIN CELLS.   Choline and docosahexaenoic acid (DHA) can help build baby's brain cells during fetal development and breastfeeding. *Choline* can be found in milk, eggs, peanuts, whole-wheat bread and beef. *DHA* is found in fish, egg yolks, poultry, meat, canola oil, walnuts and wheat germ. Encourage your partner to eat these foods during pregnancy for baby's good health. Also see the two discussions below on fish.

CHOOSE HIGH-FIBER FOODS.   Foods that are high in fiber and low in sugar and fat are good choices for a food plan. Fruits and vegetables, and whole-grain crackers and breads are excellent selections. To avoid extra calories, include foods that are high in protein but low in fat, such as skinless chicken and turkey, tuna packed in water, cod, ground turkey and lowfat (1%) or nonfat milk.

FISH CAN BE AN EXCELLENT CHOICE.   Fish can be a healthful addition to a pregnancy food plan. Fish contains omega-3 fatty acids, which may help prevent pregnancy-induced hypertension and pre-eclampsia. Omega-3 fatty acids are also good for baby's brain development. According to some studies, another benefit of eating a variety of fish is that a pregnant woman may not deliver as early as

Understanding Serving Portions of the Food Guide Pyramid

Many people today overeat because they do not understand what constitutes a "portion," as proscribed by the USDA's Food Guide Pyramid. You and your partner may believe it will be difficult for her to eat all the portions she needs for the health of your growing baby.

To learn the *correct* serving size for each of the food groups, as listed above, check out the USDA's website—www.cnpp.usda.gov—which lists serving portions. For example, a large bagel can actually be *four* to *five* grain servings!

she would have if she had not eaten fish, so babies are born with higher birth weights.

Many fish are safe to eat; most fish is low in fat and high in vitamin B, iron, zinc, selenium and copper. Many fish choices are an excellent, healthful addition to a meal plan. Good fish and shellfish choices include bass, catfish, clams, cod, crab, croaker, flounder, haddock, herring, lobster, mackerel, marlin, oysters, perch (both freshwater and ocean), orange roughy, Pacific halibut, pollack, red snapper, salmon, scallops, scrod, shrimp and sole. Other fish should be avoided; see the discussion below.

The U.S. Food and Drug Administration recommends a pregnant woman eat no more than 12 ounces of fish a week. This can be divided any way she wants—two 6-ounce servings, four 3-ounce servings or any other serving sizes that equal 12 ounces. The goal is *not* to exceed 12 ounces in any one week.

Foods to Avoid or to Eat in Moderation

BE CAREFUL WITH JUNK FOODS. If your partner is watching her calorie intake to avoid gaining unnecessary weight, you may have to stop buying foods that don't provide good nutrition. Cookies, chocolate, cake, pie, chips, candy and ice cream have lots of empty calories. It may help if you both eliminate junk food from your eating regimen. Foods we consider "junk" are usually high-calorie, high-fat foods that contain little or no nutrition for you, your partner or the growing baby. It's probably OK to eat junk food once in a while, just don't make it a regular part of your diet. You might not like the idea of eliminating these foods, but it's only for a short time. You may find you also benefit from avoiding a lot of junk food.

SOME FOODS MAY CAUSE *LISTERIOSIS*.   Some foods made from milk and foods from other sources should be avoided by a pregnant woman. They are a common source of a form of food poisoning called *listeriosis*. These foods include unpasteurized milk, any food made from unpasteurized milk, soft cheeses, such as Brie, Camembert, feta and Roquefort, undercooked poultry, undercooked meat, undercooked seafood and undercooked hot dogs. Any of these foods can contain listeriosis. Avoid the cheeses listed, and cook all meat and seafood *thoroughly* to avoid the problem.

SOME FISH TO AVOID.   Although many fish are excellent sources of nutrients, as discussed above, some should be avoided during pregnancy. Some fish are contaminated with dangerous substances as a result of man-made pollution. Studies indicate that pregnant women should not eat some kinds of fish more than once a month, including shark, swordfish, king mackerel, tilefish and tuna (fresh or frozen). Canned tuna is a little safer, but only one 6-ounce can should be eaten a week. (This must be included in the 12-ounce weekly total discussed above.)

Prenatal Vitamins Are Important

Did the doctor prescribe prenatal vitamins for your partner to take during pregnancy? Most pregnant women take a daily prenatal vitamin to meet the increased demands on their body for more vitamins and minerals while baby is growing and developing. To help your partner remember to take her prenatal vitamin, you might suggest she take it at the same time each day—for some women taking it in the evening before bed is easier on their stomach. It may help if you took *your* vitamins at the same time; you can remind one another not to skip this important step to better health. As they say, two minds are better than one!

Some freshwater fish may also be risky to eat, such as walleye, pike or lake trout. To be on the safe side, call local or state authorities for any advisories on eating freshwater fish. Parasites, bacteria, viruses and toxins can also contaminate fish. Sushi and ceviche are fish dishes that could contain viruses or parasites. Raw shellfish, if contaminated, could cause hepatitis-A, cholera or gastroenteritis. *All* raw fish should be avoided during pregnancy!

Other fish to avoid during pregnancy include some found in warm tropical waters, especially Florida, the Caribbean and Hawaii. Avoid the following "local" fish from those areas: amberjack, barracuda, bluefish, grouper, mahimahi, snapper and fresh tuna.

Is It Important When She Eats?

Researchers have found that pregnant women who eat frequent, small meals during the day may provide better nutrition to their growing babies than women who eat three large meals. Though they are eating the same amount of calories, there is a difference.

We have found that keeping the level of nutrients constant (by eating frequent, small meals) is better for fetal development than eating a large meal, then not eating again for quite a while. Three larger meals means that nutrient levels rise and fall during the day, which isn't as beneficial for the growing baby. Eating small meals frequently can also help avoid some problems associated with pregnancy, such as nausea, heartburn and indigestion.

> If your partner exercises during her pregnancy, she may also feel better if she eats small meals frequently (every 2 or 3 hours). It helps her maintain a relatively constant level of food in her system, available for use by herself and her growing baby.

As a couple, you can try to eat your meals together. Your partner's meals will be smaller, and she may have to eat earlier or later than you usually do, but with a little planning, you can do it. For example, you probably eat breakfast together, about the same time, every morning. Keep doing this. If you can't be home for dinner when she must eat, don't eat as much food as you normally do when you do eat dinner. Save some of it, and eat it when she eats her snack before bedtime. Adjustments by both of you can help you continue to share time together. And remember—it's for the good of your partner and your developing baby!

Are Food Cravings Normal?

You may be surprised by some of the weird foods your partner wants to eat. For years, comedians used "pickles and ice cream" as a craving many pregnant women had. You may find your partner's cravings are not that strange, or they may be stranger! We are unsure why women have food cravings, but many researchers believe it is caused by the hormonal changes and emotional changes that occur during pregnancy.

> ## BROWNIE POINTS
>
> Say "Yes!" to adding citrus fruit and dark, leafy greens, such as spinach, broccoli, brussels sprouts and kale, to your meal plans. They provide many of the essential nutrients your partner and your growing baby need.

For many pregnant women, food cravings are a normal part of pregnancy. A craving for a particular food can be either good or bad. If your partner craves foods that are nutritious and healthy, encourage her to eat them in moderate amounts. If she craves foods that are high in sugar and fat, and loaded with empty calories, encourage her to make more healthful choices.

PICA.   There is a condition in which pregnant women crave nonfood items, such as ice, clay, coffee grounds, cornstarch, wax and other substances. This kind of craving is called *pica,* and it isn't healthy for the woman or her baby. It can cause a variety of problems, including blocked bowels, nutritional deficiencies and severe constipation.

If your partner has these kinds of cravings, suggest she talk to the doctor about them. He or she may prescribe a supplement, usually iron, to help deal with the

> ### My Mother-in-Law Said
>
> *Pica (chewing clay, eating starch or ingesting some other nonfood item) is a way to relieve tension.*
>
> It isn't! If you notice your partner has these cravings, be sure you both discuss it with the doctor at one of her prenatal appointments.

problem. Whatever you do, don't encourage her to indulge nonfood cravings.

FLUID IS ESSENTIAL TO A HEALTHY PREGNANCY

Encourage your partner to drink a lot of fluid during pregnancy. Water is the best source; however, other fluids are acceptable. Foods and drinks that can provide fluid include vegetables, milk and milk products, meats, grain products, fruits and juices. A few of the herbal teas may be helpful for various pregnancy symptoms. See the box on herbs and botanicals beginning on page 42. It lists acceptable herbs and those that should be avoided during pregnancy.

Coffee, tea and many sodas should be avoided as fluid sources—they can contain sodium, a lot of calories and caffeine, which acts as a diuretic. If you find a low-sodium soda that doesn't contain caffeine, your partner should be able to enjoy one occasionally, but beware of the sugar content if weight gain is a concern for the mom-to-be.

Eight 8-ounce glasses of liquid a day is a good goal to work toward. Your partner can drink tap water or bottled water, but if she chooses bottled water, be sure it meets safety guidelines. Water from a municipal water supply must meet minimum government safety standards. A recent study showed that nearly 35% of all bottled water sold in the United States does *not* meet these minimum safety standards! Just because it comes from a bottle does *not* make it better. In addition, if your water comes from a well on your

Be Cautious with Caffeine

High levels of caffeine ingested by a pregnant woman—400mg a day, equal to 4 cups of tea, soda or coffee—may affect a baby's developing respiratory system. One study showed this exposure before birth might be linked to sudden infant death syndrome (SIDS). Encourage your partner to be cautious with her caffeine intake.

property, discuss it at one of your prenatal visits. Your pregnancy doctor may have some guidelines for consuming well water.

Drinking adequate amounts of fluid is important for many reasons. It enables the body to process nutrients, develop new cells, sustain blood volume and regulate body temperature—all very important during pregnancy! A woman's blood volume increases during pregnancy; drinking extra fluids helps keep up with the change. Your partner may feel better during pregnancy if she drinks more liquid than she normally does. You will note that in many of the discussions of pregnancy conditions in Chapter 3, we suggest drinking extra fluid may help relieve symptoms. In addition, extra fluid may provide other benefits, including:

✓ boosting endurance
✓ easing constipation
✓ preventing headaches
✓ helping avoid urinary-tract infections

If *you* drink extra fluid as a way to help support your partner's efforts, you may also benefit. Studies show that most people— women *and* men—do not drink enough fluid to meet their bodies' needs.

Artificial Sweeteners

Studies have not shown any harm to pregnancy from *aspartame* (Nutrasweet). The phenylalanine in aspartame contributes to phenylalanine in the diet, so if this is a problem for your partner, encourage her to avoid foods and beverages sweetened with aspartame. *Saccharin* is an artificial sweetener found in some foods and beverages; its effect on pregnancy is still being studied. As for some of the newer artificial sweeteners, we do not have enough information at this time to determine whether they are safe for your partner to use.

The best advice we can give is for your partner to avoid artificial sweeteners or to use them in moderation during pregnancy.

AN EXERCISE ROUTINE
CAN BE BENEFICIAL FOR YOU BOTH

You may be wondering if it is OK for a pregnant woman to exercise. Many medical experts agree that exercise during pregnancy is safe and beneficial for most pregnant women, if it's done properly. Exercise can help your partner deal with demands on her energy. It can improve her sleep; the better circulation fostered by exercise is beneficial for her and the baby.

IN THE DOGHOUSE

Don't ask your partner to participate in exercise activities that increase her risk of falling, such as playing a hard game of racquetball or taking a step-aerobics class.

Exercise can prepare your partner for the hard work of labor and delivery. There may be other benefits, too—one study showed women who exercise moderately during pregnancy may have a lower rate of miscarriage. Researchers believe exercise may help control some hormonal changes that lead to uterine contractions.

Your partner may be interested in exercising during her pregnancy to help her feel better and to stay in shape. Or there may be times during pregnancy when she may not want to exercise at all, especially if she experiences morning sickness or fatigue. Suggest your partner discuss exercise with the doctor at one of her first prenatal visits. A physician should be consulted *before* a pregnant woman starts exercising or when she changes her current exercise program. If you go to prenatal appointments, together you can discuss with the doctor any precautions your partner might need to take. Then you'll both know what her limits are or what precautions she may need to practice.

Use the experience of exercising together as a way to grow closer. It's fun to walk, swim, ride bicycles or exercise at the gym together. Your partner will appreciate your support, and you may appreciate the results *you* get!

What Kinds of Exercises Can We Do Together?

You may believe a pregnant woman is very limited in the type of exercise she can participate in. Not so! There are many activities that are acceptable for a mother-to-be, especially if she has been physically active before pregnancy.

Go to the gym together when you can. A moderate exercise plan will probably be best. You might consider taking an aerobics class together. They're fun, as long as everyone can work at his or her own pace.

If your club has a pool, swimming is an excellent way to get a good workout. As your partner gets bigger, she'll feel great in the water, too! Some clubs offer water aerobics classes—you can both get a good workout without stressing your joints.

> **BROWNIE POINTS**
>
> If your partner exercises during pregnancy, do it together! Make plans to walk together in the evening, to meet at the gym for a workout or take a low-impact aerobics class together.

Using various pieces of cardiovascular equipment, such as an exercise bike or a stair climber, lets you work out together. You can set the resistance or pace on your equipment to meet your particular needs, and she can do the same.

If you like to hike on the weekends, ask your partner to join you! You might want to choose easier hikes so you can enjoy them together. Avoid steep, rocky or strenuous trails because of the stress they can put on her changing body. Don't put either of you in an unsafe situation.

Bicycle riding can be fun, if your partner feels comfortable. During pregnancy, her center of gravity shifts; this might make balancing a bike more difficult for her. But if she's an experienced rider, and she has good posture and muscle control, *and* she feels confident, a bike ride can be great fun. Getting outside and enjoying the fresh air can be revitalizing. A word of caution—your partner should avoid mountain biking or any other type of extreme cycling. It might also be wise to stop biking during the third trimester, when it's harder to get on and off the bike safely.

Whatever you choose to do, do it together! Sharing the things you do during pregnancy will carry over to sharing the things you will do as parents of your new baby. For example, after baby's birth, you may find yourself buying a baby seat for your bike, and an activity will become a family one.

Some fun activities that you can enjoy together are listed below; most are considered acceptable for women of any age in a normal, low-risk pregnancy. Check out this list—you may find quite a few activities you can do together:

✓ walking
✓ swimming
✓ low-impact aerobics
✓ water aerobics
✓ stationary bicycling
✓ regular cycling (if your partner is experienced)
✓ jogging (if the mom-to-be jogged regularly before pregnancy)
✓ tennis (played moderately)
✓ yoga

If your partner is used to participating in a competitive sport, such as tennis or racquetball, she may be able to continue during her pregnancy, but expect the level at which she plays to change. The goal is not to win the game but to maintain fitness and have a good time! If you play these games together, keep this advice in mind.

Some sports activities should be *avoided* during any pregnancy. They are dangerous activities for the mother and her growing baby. Be sure your partner avoids:

✓ scuba diving
✓ water skiing
✓ surfing
✓ horseback riding
✓ downhill skiing
✓ cross-country skiing
✓ any contact sport

Regular Exercise Is Important

If a pregnant woman is going to exercise during pregnancy, after getting her doctor's OK, she needs to do it *regularly*. Irregularities in an exercise routine may have an impact on the baby's development by causing premature labor, intrauterine-growth restriction, bleeding or contractions.

Exercise Guidelines for Pregnancy

Exercise can be fun, especially when you do it together. You can do many things, as we discuss above. Follow the tips below to help your partner stay healthy and keep in good shape.

✓ Exercise should be done at least 3 times a week for 20 to 30 minutes each time.

✓ Start every exercise routine with a 5-minute warm-up, and end with a 5-minute cool-down period.

✓ Your partner (and you, too) should wear comfortable clothes that offer support, such as good athletic shoes.

✓ Drink plenty of water during exercise.

✓ A pregnant woman shouldn't exercise strenuously for more than 15 to 20 minutes without the doctor's OK.

✓ The mom-to-be's pulse shouldn't exceed 140 beats a minute.

✓ Don't exercise in hot, humid weather.

✓ Exercise during the coolest part of the day.

Benefits of Exercise

SOME POSITIVE ASPECTS TO EXERCISING. Regular exercise can help in many ways. It can help relieve a woman's backaches or prevent constipation and varicose veins. It can help an expectant mother control her weight. Exercise is good for both of you to help control moods and to provide psychological well-being. And it can help you both sleep better. In addition to strengthening muscles used in labor and delivery, exercising during pregnancy may leave a pregnant woman in better shape after delivery and help her recover more quickly in the postpartum period.

Some experts now suggest a pregnant woman who exercises in her 2nd or 3rd trimester may need more calories than the extra 300 she has added to her nutrition program. Extra nutritious snacks—one 20 to 40 minutes *before* exercising and another one soon *after* the exercise is finished—can be beneficial in replenishing calories burned during a workout. Good food choices include fruits, whole-wheat bread, pasta and cereals.

IF YOUR PARTNER EXPERIENCES SWELLING.   Any exercise that involves joint movement forces water in the tissues back into the blood and helps pump blood back to the heart. If your partner experiences swelling in her ankles or legs, exercise can help with the problem. Stationary bicycling is excellent activity to help relieve swelling in the legs.

SOME LIFESTYLE CHANGES MAY BE NECESSARY

There are many other things that can affect a pregnant woman's health, in addition to her nutrition plan and exercise routine. Cigarette smoking by the pregnant woman, her exposure to secondary smoke from others smoking, alcohol use, drug use, use of "acceptable" substances, such as herbs and botanicals—all can impact on her health and baby's health. By being aware of them, you can help make the environment safe for your partner and your growing baby. (Use of herbs and botanicals is discussed in the box beginning on page 42.)

IN THE DOGHOUSE

Going to places or participating in activities that expose your pregnant partner to secondary smoke puts her and the baby at risk.

Cigarette Smoking

A pregnant woman who smokes cigarettes can greatly affect her developing baby. Research has shown that fetal and infant mortality rates increase by more than 50% in first-time-pregnant women who smoke more than one pack of cigarettes a day.

Tobacco smoke contains many harmful substances. Inhaled cigarette smoke crosses the placenta and may reduce the fetus's oxygen supply by as much as half. Toxins in cigarette smoke narrow blood vessels, which may damage the placenta and hinder baby's growth. The problem is so serious that warnings for pregnant women appear on every cigarette package.

Substances a woman inhales when she smokes also interfere with her body's absorption of some vitamins and increase her risk of pregnancy-related complications. Smoking has been associated with specific birth defects, including cleft palate, heart defects and neural-tube defects, such as spina bifida.

Serious pregnancy complications are more common in pregnant women who smoke. The risks of developing placental abruption or placenta previa increase. The risk of miscarriage, premature rupture of membranes and fetal death or death of a baby soon after birth also rises.

If she smokes, encourage your partner to give up smoking *now*. Support her in her efforts, but don't nag. You might suggest a stop-smoking course or a support group. See other suggestions in the box below. Help her understand the impact her smoking can have on the baby.

EFFECTS OF SECONDARY SMOKE.   Even if your partner doesn't smoke, exposure to secondary smoke might cause her problems. Breathing

---

Suggestions for Helping Your Partner Quit Smoking

Quitting smoking isn't easy for anyone. It may be harder for a pregnant woman because she feels emotional about many things in her life, and smoking may seem like a way to relax. But it's bad for the developing baby if its mother smokes. Below are some hints and suggestions you might make to help your partner quit smoking.

• Occupy fingers with something, like a squeeze ball, and occupy the mouth with gum or a small helping of a low-cal snack.

• Ask your partner not to buy cigarettes; instead ask others for them (if your partner has to ask someone else for every cigarette, it might make her stop).

• Put any money saved not buying cigarettes into a jar, and use it to splurge together on a nice meal or to buy something for the baby.

• Give your partner a baby bootie or make a copy of baby's ultrasound picture, and ask her to carry it with her as a reminder of why she doesn't want to smoke.

• Urge your partner to call you or someone else close to her when she thinks she needs a cigarette.

someone else's cigarette smoke could increase her risk of giving birth to a low-birthweight baby, which isn't healthy for the baby.

If you or others close to you smoke, significant changes may be necessary. Smoking outside or away from home may *not* be the answer. Cigarette smoke produces microscopic particles that are carcinogenic (cancer causing). These particles can be found on hair, skin and clothes of smokers, and are stirred up every time the person moves. They float into the air and can be breathed in by anyone who is near. Even if a person goes outside to smoke or smokes somewhere else, these unwanted particles can be brought into the environment.

For the good health of your baby and your partner (*and* for your own good health), try to give up smoking now. Do not allow others to smoke and then come into your home. If you can't stop smoking, you

---

Using Herbal Supplements and Botanicals during Pregnancy

More than 40% of the U.S. population uses some type of herbal or botanical preparation to treat ailments. There are over 400 different herbs and botanicals available today—many are used to treat a variety of problems. They are sold as tablets, capsules, tinctures, teas and extracts in health-food stores, pharmacies and other outlets.

Many people believe that because substances are considered "natural," these products are safe to take at any time. However, this is not the case. Some herbs and botanicals are OK; others are not. Before your partner takes *anything*, she should check with the doctor. Although you both may believe an herbal drug can help a woman deal with morning sickness, premature labor or other pregnancy conditions, it might actually cause problems.

One issue with herbs and botanicals is that most haven't been thoroughly tested nor have they been proved safe for use during pregnancy. Some can be very dangerous to a pregnant woman or her growing baby, so be sure you check whether an herb is safe to use during pregnancy *before* your partner uses it!

Herbal Teas

Herbal teas may be considered safer than other herbs and botanicals because they are used in a diluted strength. Many herbal teas are sold

(continued on next page)

(continued from previous page)
in grocery stores; others are harder to find and need to be purchased at a health-food store.

Some herbal teas can help relieve various pregnancy discomforts. This can make herbal tea a good alternative to coffee or regular tea. The herbal teas discussed below may help relieve certain pregnancy problems and are safe to use during pregnancy:

- chamomile—aids digestion
- dandelion—helps with swelling and can soothe an upset stomach
- ginger root—helps with nausea and nasal congestion
- nettle leaf—rich in calcium, iron and other vitamins and minerals
- peppermint—relieves gas pains and calms the stomach
- red raspberry—helps with nausea

Other herbs and herbal teas are *not* safe to use during pregnancy because they could harm your developing baby. Herbs and teas to *avoid* during pregnancy include:

* blue or black cohosh * pennyroyal leaf * yarrow * goldenseal * feverfew * psillium seed * mugwort * comfrey * coltsfoot * juniper * rue * tansy * cottonroot bark * sage (in large amounts) * senna * cascara sagrada * buckthorn * male fern * slippery elm * squaw vine * St. John's wort * gingko * echinacea * safflower * rosemary * sassafras * ephedra * willow bark * fenugreek * dong quai *

may have to take some unusual measures to avoid subjecting your partner, and later your newborn baby, to the negative effects of cigarette smoke. Consider taking a shower, washing your hair and putting on clean clothes after you smoke a cigarette, to avoid exposing your partner and developing fetus to the harmful effects of secondary smoke.

Alcohol Use during Pregnancy

When your partner drinks alcohol during pregnancy, so does your baby—the more your partner drinks, the more the baby "drinks." A developing baby may be harmed by an alcohol level that has little apparent effect on an adult. A fetus cannot metabolize alcohol as quickly as an adult, so alcohol remains in its system longer. Alcohol use by a pregnant woman can carry considerable risk to her developing fetus.

Moderate use of alcohol has been linked to a higher rate of miscarriage and spina bifida.

The best advice we can give is for a pregnant woman to avoid *all* alcohol during pregnancy. This may sound drastic, but it's the only way a woman can be sure she protects her growing baby from any effects from alcohol. Drinking as little as two drinks a day has been associated with various problems, including fetal-alcohol exposure (FAE) and fetal-alcohol syndrome (FAS). Both are characterized by abnormal fetal development.

Taking drugs with alcohol increases the risk of damaging the fetus. Drugs that cause the greatest concern include analgesics, antidepressants and anticonvulsants. Other substances, which you might not think of as being "alcohol," may contain alcohol. Various over-the-counter cough and cold remedies and some mouthwashes contain alcohol—as much as 25% of the preparation!

Encourage your partner to avoid all alcohol during her entire pregnancy. If necessary, you may choose to avoid it, too. As with changes in your nutrition and exercise plans, sharing this goal can be good for your relationship and for each of you individually. Remember, it's for the good health of your baby.

Drug Use

Drug use can greatly affect a pregnancy. A woman who uses drugs may have more pregnancy complications because of her lifestyle. These complications include nutritional deficiencies, anemia, preeclampsia and fetal-growth restriction.

If your partner uses drugs, even if it's only occasionally, encourage her to stop now! Your baby's life is at risk. Below is a discussion of various substances that are harmful to a growing baby.

✓ *Marijuana* use during pregnancy can cause problems in a child in later life, including attention-deficit disorders, memory problems and impaired decision-making ability.

✓ *Central-nervous-system stimulants,* such as amphetamines, are associated with an increase in cardiovascular defects, signs of withdrawal, poor feeding, seizures and other problems in a baby.

✓ *Tranquilizers,* such as benzodiazepines (Valium® and Librium®), are associated with an increase in birth defects.

✓ *Narcotics use,* such as morphine, Demerol®, heroin and codeine, can result in pre-eclampsia, preterm labor, fetal-growth problems and narcotic withdrawal in the baby following birth. The incidence of sudden-infant-death syndrome (SIDS) is 10 times higher among babies born to mothers who use narcotics during pregnancy than to babies whose mothers did not.

✓ *Mind-altering drugs,* including LSD, mescaline, hashish, peyote, PCP and angel dust, are believed to cause abnormal development in human babies, although this has not been definitely proved.

✓ *Cocaine* use complicates a pregnancy because a user may eat or drink very little, with serious consequences for a developing fetus. Cocaine use has been linked with miscarriage, preterm labor, bleeding complications, placental abruption and congenital defects. Cocaine can damage the developing baby as early as 3 days after conception!

**MEMORABLE MOMENTS
FROM DR. DAD**

Kate and Dave came together to her first prenatal appointment; Dave seemed quite interested in, and connected to, the pregnancy. He wanted to help Kate in any way he could. During our conversation, Kate asked me questions about nutrition and exercise; she exercised regularly and wanted to know if she could continue. I applauded her interest and encouraged her to continue her walking and low-impact aerobics. I commented that exercise was safe and good to do during pregnancy, and healthy nutrition was certainly a goal to strive for. I also said exercise is a healthy habit to get into, and paying attention to what a pregnant woman eats benefits her baby.

At that point, Dave asked if it would be OK to exercise together with Kate. I heartily endorsed it. He also told Kate that he had been thinking about a better eating plan for himself and said he would help plan meals and do some of the cooking while she was pregnant. The end result? A healthy Kate and a healthy baby.

And Dave came through the pregnancy 23 pounds lighter and in better shape!

3

Ways to Support Your Pregnant Partner

As pregnancy progresses, you will find many opportunities to show your partner you care about her and your growing baby. She needs lots of support from you. It's pretty hard to go through a pregnancy without someone close to lean on—your help and continued interest demonstrate to her that you are concerned about her health and welfare, and the baby's, too. Doing whatever is necessary to support your partner may be one of the best gifts you will ever give your child.

Your effort during these months should involve more than just being sympathetic to your partner's discomforts. In this chapter, we cover many of the physical conditions and complaints that may accompany a woman's pregnancy. In each description, we offer you suggestions on ways to provide for your partner's comfort and well-being.

Chapter Focus

In this chapter, we discuss morning sickness, heartburn, fatigue and many other common discomforts women have during pregnancy. We explain what a condition is and provide suggestions for ways you can help your partner deal with that particular situation.

We also offer some hints and tips on ways to make your partner's life easier by helping out with shopping, household chores and making your environment a safe one for the pregnant woman. We hope these tips will make pregnancy a happy experience for you both.

COMMON DISCOMFORTS
AND CONDITIONS IN PREGNANCY

This section contains discussions of many of the changes a woman might experience during pregnancy. Some cause the mom-to-be some discomfort. Others are merely changes that you should be aware of. As you can see, being pregnant causes a woman's body to change in many ways. It's not only her tummy that is growing and changing!

We may go into a lot of detail about a particular condition in the following discussions. This information is provided to give you a better understanding of the situation. We list the terms in alphabetical order so you can find them easily. You might want to check out only those your partner experiences, or you may choose to read about all the conditions.

Backache
SITUATION FOR YOUR PARTNER.   An aching back often occurs as a woman's abdomen gets bigger and changes her center of gravity. Pain may occur after walking a lot, standing, bending, lifting or exercising; it may also occur just because a woman is pregnant.

SOLUTION FOR YOU.   A back rub from you can help relieve the discomfort of a sore back. Or apply heat or cold to the area; both are safe during pregnancy. You might also take over some of the chores that require your partner to stand, bend or lift, such as washing the dishes, vacuuming, carrying laundry or cleaning the bathroom.

Bleeding Gums
SITUATION FOR YOUR PARTNER.   Pregnancy can cause your partner's gums to be sore, to bleed or to swell because of hormonal changes. Gums are more susceptible to irritation and may bleed more often with flossing or brushing.

SOLUTION FOR YOU.   Encourage your partner to brush her teeth 2 or 3 times a day and floss at least once a day to help control the problem. Regular dental checkups during pregnancy and taking care of any dental problem as soon as it arises will also help her avoid discomfort. Dental visits should *not* be avoided by a pregnant woman!

Body-Temperature Changes
SITUATION FOR YOUR PARTNER.   A woman's metabolism may increase during pregnancy because her body uses more energy. Pregnancy hormones also elevate body temperature. Both of these situations may cause your partner to feel overheated or hot.

SOLUTION FOR YOU.   Try to be considerate of this change if the mother-to-be complains about how uncomfortable she is and you feel fine. If she needs the window open, and you feel cool, put on a sweater.

Breast Changes

SITUATION FOR YOUR PARTNER. Many changes occur in the breasts during pregnancy. After about 8 weeks, it's normal for your partner's breasts to start getting larger, lumpy or nodular. They may also

BROWNIE POINTS

Make your partner feel special whenever you can. Bring home flowers, send her a card or call her on the phone during the day to tell her you were thinking about her and the baby.

be very sensitive; tenderness, tingling or soreness of the breasts early in pregnancy is common. You may notice the areola, which surrounds the nipple, also turns brown or red-brown and may get larger during pregnancy. Most women gain between 1 and 1-1/2 pounds in *each* breast by the time baby is born.

SOLUTION FOR YOU. Be careful of her breasts during intimate moments. Bumping or jarring them can cause pain. You might suggest she buy a maternity bra to provide needed support as her breasts grow larger.

Constipation

SITUATION FOR YOUR PARTNER. It's common for a woman to become constipated due to a slowdown in the movement of food through her gastrointestinal system. She may also take iron supplements, or her prenatal vitamins may contain iron. Many pregnant women experience irregular bowel habits and hemorrhoids when they are constipated.

SOLUTION FOR YOU. Increasing fluid intake and exercising 3 or 4 times a week may help if your partner experiences the problem. Encourage her to drink a lot of water every day. You may want to exercise with her, too. Some juices, such as prune juice or apple juice, or taking a mild laxative, such as milk of magnesia, Metamucil and Colace, may offer some relief. High-fiber foods, such as bran and prunes, can help relieve constipation. Encourage her to eat them.

Cravings

SITUATION FOR YOUR PARTNER.   Many women experience food cravings during pregnancy. When they crave something, they often want it *now!* Some cravings may seem very strange to you. Researchers believe cravings are caused by hormonal changes and emotional changes that occur during pregnancy.

SOLUTION FOR YOU.   If your partner craves nutritious foods, that's OK. She can probably eat them in moderate amounts. If she craves junk food, try to promote healthier choices. If your partner craves nonfood items, called *pica,* as discussed in Chapter 2, suggest she talk to her doctor about them. She may need a supplement, usually iron, which her doctor can prescribe.

My Mother-in-Law Said

If a pregnant woman craves foods that are high in vitamin C, she's carrying a girl. If she craves meat, it's going to be a boy.

There's no medical indication that any food cravings a woman experiences means the baby is one sex or the other.

Emotional Changes

SITUATION FOR YOUR PARTNER. You may notice that your partner cries at the slightest thing, daydreams or has mood swings. Her emotions are influenced by her changing hormones, which can cause these changes.

SOLUTION FOR YOU.   Try to be understanding when mood swings occur. When your partner reacts in a way that is not typical of her, try not to get angry or to overreact. If she's inattentive to you, she may be daydreaming about the baby. Ask for her attention. If she cries over something insignificant, be sympathetic, or at the least try to be understanding. Don't take it personally or get upset.

Exhaustion and Fatigue

SITUATION FOR YOUR PARTNER.   During the first part of your partner's pregnancy, all she may want to do is sleep! Feeling overly tired and not being able to get enough rest is normal. Fatigue is one of the first signs of pregnancy, and energy lows are not unusual. For most women, fatigue is the worst early in pregnancy, then it gets better. But it may recur throughout pregnancy.

SOLUTION FOR YOU.   Let your partner take it easy and rest when she can or when she feels she needs to. Encourage her to watch her diet and to drink lots of fluids. High-fat foods and dehydration can worsen the problem. Suggest she avoid sugar because it can also make fatigue worse.

If your partner can't sleep enough at night to make her feel rested, it may help her to nap during the day. Let her know you'll do some household chores so she can take it easy. Regular exercise can also help a pregnant woman feel better. Suggest taking a walk together after dinner, or do a workout videotape (one for pregnant women is best) together early in the evening. Keep your bedroom cool—70F (21.1C) is about the highest temperature for comfortable sleeping.

BROWNIE POINTS

Make a date with your partner for a night free of cooking and cleaning up. Order take-out food and watch a video, or go out for dinner, followed by a stroll in the evening air.

Be understanding when your partner doesn't have the energy to get out of bed at times. One of her main goals in life may be getting enough rest. Support her in her efforts—she really does feel exhausted!

Food Aversions

SITUATION FOR YOUR PARTNER.   Some foods may make your partner sick to her stomach. This is common during pregnancy. Pregnancy hormones have a significant impact on the gastrointestinal tract, which can affect a woman's reaction to certain foods. Don't be surprised if she can't stand the sight of some food she normally loves.

SOLUTION FOR YOU.   If a food you enjoy is one that nauseates the mom-to-be, don't ask her to prepare it or even to sit with you when you eat it. You could prepare it yourself when she's not around, or eat it when you are out, such as at lunch, when your partner isn't with you. When you're finished, clean up your pans and dishes. Just washing up the cooking utensils may make a pregnant woman feel ill.

Forgetfulness

SITUATION FOR YOUR PARTNER.   Being forgetful may not seem as though it could be related to pregnancy, but it can be. Some researchers believe increased hormone levels are at play. Fatigue and sleep deprivation may also be partially responsible.

SOLUTION FOR YOU.   You may have to make lists for your partner to remind her of obligations, errands or important events. If you approach the situation with humor, your solution is more likely to be accepted. And who knows—it could become an important aspect of your lives together.

Frequent Urination

SITUATION FOR YOUR PARTNER.   One of the first signs of pregnancy is frequent urination. This problem continues off and on throughout pregnancy. It usually lessens during the second trimester, then returns during the third trimester, when the growing baby puts pressure on the bladder.

SOLUTION FOR YOU.   Listen when the mother-to-be says she has to go to the bathroom. She *really* does have to go! When you're out and about together, plan to make frequent potty stops. It also helps to know where bathrooms are located, so you can find them easily when you need them. Grocery stores, drugstores and shopping malls usually have public facilities. If your partner needs to go to the bathroom and you don't see one handy, *ask* someone in the store if a restroom is available to use.

Headaches

SITUATION FOR YOUR PARTNER.   A woman may experience more tension headaches during pregnancy due to sleep disturbances, nausea and vomiting, and stress (emotional and physical). These may decrease during the second and third trimesters of pregnancy as her body (and mind) adjust to pregnancy.

SOLUTION FOR YOU.   It's good to avoid unnecessary medication during pregnancy. Medicine-free ways to relieve headaches that you can do together include deep-breathing exercises and relaxation techniques, applying an ice pack to the back of her head or nape of her neck and making sure the mom-to-be gets enough sleep in a quiet place.

If your partner's headaches don't go away using these techniques, suggest she take regular or extra-strength acetaminophen (Tylenol). If this doesn't help, ask her to discuss the situation with the doctor.

Heartburn

SITUATION FOR YOUR PARTNER.   Heartburn is a burning discomfort felt behind the lower part of the breastbone; it is one of the most common complaints during pregnancy. It may begin early in pregnancy, although it generally becomes more severe as pregnancy progresses. Heartburn is caused by reflux (regurgitation) of stomach contents into the esophagus. It may become more of a problem during the third trimester when the expanding uterus crowds your partner's stomach and intestines.

SOLUTION FOR YOU.   Some foods can cause the problem, such as rich or spicy foods. If you love them and they cause your partner problems, avoid eating them in her presence and don't ask her to prepare them only for you! She should also avoid eating before bedtime—it's a good idea for you, too. When lying down, her head and shoulders should be elevated; raising the head of your bed might help. Antacids may provide relief; package directions relating to pregnancy should be followed. Amphojel, Gelusil, milk of magnesia and Maalox can be used with moderation. See the box that follows *Indigestion,* page 56, for precautions regarding some medications.

Hemorrhoids

SITUATION FOR YOUR PARTNER.   Hemorrhoids are dilated blood vessels around the anus or up inside the anus. A pregnant woman may get hemorrhoids because her body tissues lose some elasticity. In addition, the increased weight and size of the enlarging uterus causes pressure and blocks blood flow in the pelvic area, which encourages hemorrhoid formation. Hemorrhoids can itch, bleed and cause pain.

SOLUTION FOR YOU.   Try to be sympathetic if your partner suffers from hemorrhoids. If they make her life miserable, suggest she discuss the situation with the doctor. Many measures can help relieve discomfort.

Indigestion

SITUATION FOR YOUR PARTNER.   Indigestion refers to the body's inability to digest food or difficulty digesting food. This condition may occur during pregnancy, even if the woman has not suffered with it before.

Pepcid® AC (for acid control) and *Tagamet HB®* (for heartburn relief) are two over-the-counter medications advertised to relieve indigestion and heartburn. However, we advise women *not* to use these products during pregnancy, except in rare cases. If your partner has problems and has used these products in the past, encourage her to discuss their use during pregnancy with the doctor, who will decide whether these products are acceptable for her to use now. Discourage her from starting these products without first consulting the physician.

SOLUTION FOR YOU.   It's always good to try nonmedication solutions first. Suggest your partner eat small, frequent meals of low-fat foods, which may be more easily digested than high-fat food. Foods that cause problems, such as rich or spicy foods, should also be avoided. She should also avoid eating before bedtime. When she lies down, her head and shoulders should be elevated; raising the head of your bed might help. Suggest she avoid

carbonated beverages. Be sure you have noncarbonated ones available, such as fruit juices.

Itching
SITUATION FOR YOUR PARTNER.   Itching may occur during pregnancy;
about 20% of all pregnant women experience it. It usually occurs later
in pregnancy. As the uterus grows and fills the pelvis, abdominal skin
and muscles stretch to accommodate it. This stretching of the skin
causes abdominal itching in many women.

SOLUTION FOR YOU.   There's not a lot you can do for your partner
to help relieve itching other than offering to rub lotion on itchy areas she can't reach. Use a body moisturizer, or if it's hot and humid,
a cornstarch-based powder may offer more relief. Avoid talcum
powder because researchers believe it may irritate bronchial tubes.
Various creams, such as hydrocortisone cream, may be OK to use;
your partner needs to check first with the doctor. Encourage her not
to scratch because it could result in more discomfort.

Leg Cramps
SITUATION FOR YOUR PARTNER.   Leg cramps, also called *charley
horses,* can be a pain during pregnancy, especially at night. A
cramp is a spasm in two sets of muscles that forces the foot to
point involuntarily and is characterized by a sharp, grabbing pain
in the calf.

SOLUTION FOR YOU.   Stretching muscles helps relieve cramps. Help
your partner when she has a cramp by gently pulling the upper part
of her foot upward while she presses her knee. (It may be hard for
her to reach her foot because of her growing tummy.) Massage her
legs at the end of the day or whenever your partner feels it would
help. Suggest your partner avoid soft drinks, snack foods and
processed foods that are high in phosphates, which can contribute
to the problem. Standing for long periods of time may cause leg
cramps. Help out with tasks around the house that your partner

normally does that involve standing for any length of time, such as ironing or doing the dishes.

Migraine Headaches

SITUATION FOR YOUR PARTNER. A migraine headache is characterized by severe throbbing pain aggravated by physical activity. Some women who regularly experience migraines when they are not pregnant do not suffer from them during pregnancy. Others have worse migraine headaches, especially in the first trimester. For some, the 2nd and 3rd trimesters are migraine-free. If your partner has had migraine headaches before pregnancy, suggest she discuss them at her first prenatal visit.

SOLUTION FOR YOU. If the mom-to-be experiences a migraine for the first time during pregnancy, she may want to try to deal with it first without medicine. She can lie in a darkened room with a cold compress on her forehead. Relaxation methods, such as listening to relaxation tapes, doing deep-breathing exercises or practicing meditation/yoga exercises, may offer relief. Help your partner avoid things that might trigger a migraine, such as aged cheese, cured meat, chocolate, caffeine, cigarette or cigar smoke, bright lights, stress or disruptions in sleeping or eating patterns. If these measures don't help, she should talk with the doctor, who will prescribe the safest medication available. Your partner should *not* take any medication, other than acetaminophen, for any headache without discussing it first with her physician.

Morning Sickness or Nausea and Vomiting

SITUATION FOR YOUR PARTNER. An early symptom of pregnancy for many women is nausea, with or without vomiting; it is often called *morning sickness*. The problem doesn't occur only in the morning; it may be experienced at any time of day, and it may last all day long. Researchers believe the problem may be caused by an imbalance in vitamin B$_6$. The condition usually begins around week 6 and lasts until week 12 or 13, when it starts to subside. Sometimes it can last all through pregnancy.

Morning sickness can cause a pregnant woman to feel ill, to avoid food or drink, to lose weight and to miss work. It is such a real condition that if morning sickness causes a woman to be absent from her job, the Family and Medical Leave Act (FMLA) states the woman does *not* need a doctor's note verifying the problem. Nausea/vomiting is classified as a "chronic condition" of pregnancy.

SOLUTION FOR YOU.   Morning sickness can be debilitating, so be sympathetic and try to help out in any way you can. There

A pill to help relieve the symptoms of morning sickness is now available; it is called *Bendectin*. If your partner has a great deal of trouble with morning sickness, suggest she ask the doctor about it.

are some things you can do to help your partner with the discomfort she experiences. *Before* she gets out of bed in the morning, bring your partner a snack, such as dry crackers, dry toast or rice cakes, to help settle her stomach. Make changes in the environment to help your partner avoid things that trigger her nausea, such as odors, movement or noise. Help the mom-to-be keep up her fluid intake—fluids may be easier to handle than solids and they help her avoid dehydration. Offer to get her water or something else to drink whenever she needs it or wants it. You might consider buying her some "pregnancy lollipops" to help deal with the problem. Pops are now available to help reduce nausea and dry mouth, and they come in a variety of flavors. Ask about them at your drugstore or food market.

Grate some fresh ginger for your partner to eat or to steep as tea. It's a natural remedy for nausea. Or cut up a fresh lemon for her to suck on when she feels nauseous. Be sure your partner gets enough rest. Watch TV or read in another room when she wants to sleep. If she normally prepares meals, offer to cook for a while because her sense of smell may be extra sensitive, which can contribute to her nausea. If a certain food that you eat makes her sick, don't eat it in front of her. Buy her a motion-sickness bracelet or wristband; it can help relieve nausea. Suggest to your partner that she eat small, frequent meals. A full stomach, or an empty one, may make her feel sick. Don't even talk about food—just the mere mention could make her sick.

Let her know you sympathize with the discomfort she is feeling, and tell her all she has to do is to ask you for help, and you'll be there. Let her know she needs to be as specific as she can about ways you can help her. Keep communication open between you.

Nosebleeds
SITUATION FOR YOUR PARTNER.   Occasional nosebleeds are not uncommon in some pregnant women. Pregnancy hormones circulating through the body may contribute to the problem.

SOLUTION FOR YOU.   If nosebleeds are a problem for your partner, buy a humidifier for your home, especially if you live in a dry climate. Be sure it's in good working order so it keeps the environment comfortable. A little petroleum jelly in her nostrils can also relieve dryness, so make sure it's available.

Round-Ligament Pain
SITUATION FOR YOUR PARTNER.   Round ligaments are attached to either side of the uterus. As your partner's uterus gets bigger, quick movements can stretch the ligaments and hurt; pain can be felt on a woman's sides, below the bellybutton. This is not harmful to your partner or your baby, but it can be uncomfortable.

SOLUTION FOR YOU.   Help the mom-to-be up when necessary to avoid movements that might cause her pain. Sometimes rapid movements can result in an increase in pain. Take things slowly.

Sciatic-Nerve Pain
SITUATION FOR YOUR PARTNER.   Your partner may experience an excruciating pain from the buttocks down the back or the side of her leg; this is sciatic-nerve pain. The sciatic nerve runs behind the uterus in the pelvis to the legs; pressure on the nerve from the growing uterus is believed to cause the pain. Pain may occur when your partner stands, walks or sits down, and it may occur more frequently as pregnancy progresses.

SOLUTION FOR YOU.   Do not allow your partner to do any heavy lifting. Standing may also contribute to the situation, so take over her tasks that involve standing. If she must stand for any length of time, provide some object she can rest the toes of the affected leg on that is 3 to 4 inches off the ground, such as a thick book (the phone book or a dictionary is good for this task!). This helps relieve pressure on the sciatic nerve. Encourage the mom-to-be to lie on her side, on the opposite side of the pain, if she experiences sciatic pain. You may want to try some of the massage techniques for relieving sciatic pain found on page 107.

Sexual Desire

SITUATION FOR YOUR PARTNER.   It's common for a woman's sexual desire to change during pregnancy. Some women experience a decrease in desire. Some experience a heightened sexual desire—an increase tends to occur during the second trimester.

SOLUTION FOR YOU.   Be patient and understanding about how your partner feels about sex during this time. Discuss the situation with her, and work out a plan that suits both of you. You may have to use your imaginations to devise ways to enjoy sexual intimacy as her body grows bigger. Be creative, and don't take it all too seriously.

Skin Changes

SITUATION FOR YOUR PARTNER.   Most women experience some changes in their skin while pregnant. Some women have very dry skin; some have oilier skin and pimples. Some lucky women find their skin becomes less oily and softer. Other skin changes include brown patches on the face, called *chloasma* or *mask of pregnancy,* redness of the palms, called *palmar erythema,* red elevations on the skin of the neck and upper chest, called *vascular spiders,* and the appearance of a dark vertical line on the lower abdomen, called the *linea nigra.* Some women find they grow new moles, or existing ones may change. These changes are all due to the hormones of pregnancy.

SOLUTION FOR YOU.   Luckily, changes to the skin do not usually cause concern or problems for a pregnant woman; however, growth or a change in a mole should *always* be brought to a doctor's attention. Be supportive of your partner if she experiences skin changes. Sometimes they are hard to deal with because they make a pregnant woman feel self-conscious. Let her know you think she's beautiful. Skin changes are often temporary, and many will disappear after the baby's birth. If your partner has extremely dry skin, offer to rub lotions and creams into her sensitive skin. If she has acne, suggest she discuss the situation with the doctor, who may prescribe some special creams she can use on her skin.

Stretch Marks

SITUATION FOR YOUR PARTNER.   Stretch marks are areas of stretched skin that may become discolored. Not every woman gets them, and for those who do, they can range from very few to many. Marks usually occur on the abdomen as the growing uterus stretches skin; they can also occur on the breasts, hips or buttocks. Stretch marks usually fade and won't be as noticeable after pregnancy.

SOLUTION FOR YOU.   Stretch marks often accompany pregnancy. There isn't much that can be done about them, but you can suggest your partner ask the doctor if there are any creams or lotions that she can use to help deal with the problem.

Swelling

SITUATION FOR YOUR PARTNER.   A pregnant woman's body produces as much as 50% more blood and fluid to meet a developing baby's needs. Some of this extra fluid can leak into her body tissues. When her enlarging uterus pushes on pelvic veins, blood flow in the lower part of the body is partially blocked. This pushes fluid into your partner's legs and feet, causing swelling. Her hands may also swell. Foods that contain large amounts of sodium, such as salty foods, processed foods, pickles, fast foods and carbonated beverages, may contribute to the problem.

SOLUTION FOR YOU. Be sympathetic when your partner bemoans the fact she can't get her shoes on or her rings won't fit. Buy her a pretty chain she can wear around her neck to hold her rings. You can also help out by massaging her legs and feet or her hands and arms. Provide pillows to put under her legs when she lies down to rest. Encourage her to lie on her side (left is best) to help relieve the problem. Exercise together—it can help prevent swelling.

Varicose Veins

SITUATION FOR YOUR PARTNER. Varicose veins (varices) are dilated blood vessels that fill with blood. They usually occur in the legs but also appear in the birth canal and in the vulva, or they can be seen as hemorrhoids. For some women, varicose veins are only a blemish or purple-blue spot on the legs. They cause little or no discomfort, except in the evening. For other women, varices are bulging veins that require compression stockings during the day and elevation of the legs at the end of the day.

> **One Way to Help Avoid Swelling**
>
> If your partner experiences common swelling of her hands and feet, you may have to skip some of the foods you both normally love. High on the list of places to avoid are Chinese-food restaurants because they often use a lot of monosodium glutamate (MSG) in their food preparation. Sodium is one of the main culprits that contributes to swelling. So to help your partner avoid added discomfort, you might want to avoid eating Chinese food. Or you might try to find some that do not use MSG in food preparation; they do exist!

SOLUTION FOR YOU. Make sure pillows are at hand to elevate your partner's legs when she relaxes. If she needs to wear compression hose, they may be easier to get on *before* she gets out of bed in the morning. In this situation, be sure she has the hose to put on before she gets up. You may also need to help her put them on.

Weight Gain

SITUATION FOR YOUR PARTNER. A pregnant woman is expected to gain weight during pregnancy; it's necessary for the baby's good

Products to Help
Relieve Some Pregnancy Discomforts

Does your medicine cabinet contain the basic necessities that you'll need in the months ahead to help you and your partner cope with some of the common discomforts discussed in this section? Is it filled with items you may need during pregnancy? It's a good idea to have some supplies handy to help relieve symptoms. Below is a list of items commonly found at the drugstore or grocery store that you might want to stock up on now.

• acetaminophen—helps relieve headaches and other minor aches and pains (Tylenol)

• antacids—good for dealing with heartburn; liquids may offer greater relief because they also coat the esophagus (Amphojel, Gelusil, Maalox, milk of magnesia)

• anti-itch preparations—if itching becomes a problem, these can help relieve discomfort (calamine lotion, Benadryl)

• body lotion—good for back rubs, to deal with dry skin and to relieve itching

• cough medicine—if your partner gets a cold or experiences any coughing (Robitussin)

• decongestants—help deal with nasal stuffiness (chlorpheniramine, Sudafed)

• diarrhea preparation—for those instances when your partner gets the flu or eats something that causes diarrhea (Kaopectate, Imodium)

• foot lotion—good for foot massages

• hemorrhoid cream, ointment or pads—when your partner needs relief from hemorrhoidal itching or pain (Anusol, Preparation H, Tucks)

• minipads—to protect against mishaps with leaking urine and for vaginal discharge

• motion-sickness bands—these wristbands can help relieve the nausea associated with morning sickness

• pimple cream—over-the-counter topical acne medication may help your partner deal with skin breakouts

• stool softeners—to deal with constipation (Colace)

• throat lozenges—for relief of a sore throat or a dry throat (Sucrets)

• witch hazel—put on cotton balls or cotton pads and apply to hemorrhoids health. An average-weight woman should gain between 25 and 35 pounds during a normal pregnancy. This may sound like a lot of weight, but the woman doesn't gain it all. Total weight gain includes the weight of the baby, amniotic fluid, placenta, increased fluid volume and breast enlargement. A woman gains only about 7 to 12 pounds of the total weight.

SOLUTION FOR YOU. Help your partner watch her weight by encouraging good nutrition and moderate exercise, but *don't* act as the "weight police." And be careful about making jokes or rude comments about your partner's changing body and weight distribution. Either can be hurtful.

YOUR PARTNER'S BODY IMAGE

It's obvious to nearly everyone—a woman's body changes a great deal during pregnancy. Your partner's feelings about her growing body are very complex. Just about every pregnant woman feels unattractive at times during her pregnancy. Your partner may have many different feelings about the changes she experiences. It's normal. And the fact that a woman is expected to gain weight as the months pass can add to the situation, especially if she has watched her weight closely in the past. But there are some things you can do to help the mom-to-be feel good about herself.

TELL HER SHE'S BEAUTIFUL. It's important to tell your partner you think she's beautiful at this time. She needs to hear from you that you find her attractive; many men *do* find a pregnant woman's rounded,

If your pregnant partner tells you she feels large, cumbersome and awkward, she is expressing feelings pregnant women have felt for thousands of years.

How do we know? The ancient Egyptians had a goddess of pregnancy called *Taweret*. Statues show her as half-woman, half-hippopotamus! That may convey how women felt about being pregnant 3,000 years ago. Times don't seem to have changed much!

full body appealing! The pregnancy "glow," which may in part be caused by the happiness, excitement and anticipation of the coming baby, often adds to a woman's beauty. If this may not be completely true for you, a little white lie will go a long way in helping your partner feel good about the changes she is experiencing.

IN THE DOGHOUSE

Don't comment on your partner's physical size, such as mentioning how big she's getting or informing her that her feet are gigantic.

FOCUS ON GOOD HEALTH.   Talk to your partner about having a healthy baby. Reassure her that gaining an adequate amount of weight is important to ensure the good health of the baby. Help her separate "pregnant" and "fat."

PAMPER HER.   Suggest your partner get a facial or a pedicure and a manicure. Buy her a pretty maternity outfit, or if you don't feel com-

---

MEMORABLE MOMENTS
FROM DR. DAD

Toward the end of Ian and Megan's pregnancy, they came in together for one of their last prenatal visits before their baby was born. They were laughing, and I asked them to share the joke. Megan showed me her left hand just like a newly engaged woman. I looked but saw only a small gold band on her finger and looked at her questioningly. Ian explained that she was wearing a "new," larger wedding band because her hands were so swollen she was unable to wear her engagement and wedding rings. He laughed when he told me he bought the new ring at a local discount store, and this one was much less expensive than the ones he bought before. At only $3.99, he said he could buy her three or four more, but Megan said she was quite pleased with this one. Megan further stated that although this was kind of a funny situation, it was a relief for her to be able to wear a wedding band.

fortable shopping for maternity clothes, buy her flowers, a CD or a piece of jewelry, or send her a sentimental card. Make her feel special.

DON'T COMPARE HER TO ANYONE ELSE.   Many people don't like to be compared to others; this can be especially true of a pregnant woman. Her pregnancy is unique to her, so don't comment on her friend's pregnant body or even compare your partner to her prepregnancy size.

ENCOURAGE HER TO TALK TO YOU.   Let her know you are available to listen to her thoughts about how she feels about her changing body. Reassure her that her feelings are normal.

UNDERSTAND EMOTIONS CAN PLAY A PART.   Remember your partner may be very emotional at this time, so be prepared if she reacts in an unexpected way to a comment you make or a suggestion you offer her about her appearance.

OFFER YOUR PARTNER YOUR SUPPORT

There are a lot of ways you can offer your support to your pregnant partner. From helping her deal with her discomforts to helping her deal with her changing body, be there for her. You can also let her know how important she and your growing baby are to you by helping out whenever you can, doing tasks that make her life easier and making her environment safe.

Help Out around the House
Do you normally relax when you get home and leave running the house to your partner? Now's the time to assume the responsibility of doing some of the tasks around the house to help your partner. Your assistance can allow the mom-to-be to relax more and to avoid unsafe situations or ones that could tire her or cause her stress.

Any chores you do to reduce your partner's stress and fatigue help you out; when the mom-to-be feels happy and healthy, you'll feel good, too. Offer to help, and ask what your partner would like you to do. Be aware that she may still want control of this part of her life. Below is a list of some things you might offer to do.

✓ Do the vacuuming. Sometimes the strain of pushing a vacuum cleaner around the house can cause fatigue.

✓ Clean the bathroom, including the bathtub. Some of the cleaners may make her feel ill. Bending over and reaching down into the tub can cause back pain, and it can be pretty uncomfortable, too.

✓ Empty the dishwasher. Bending over and lifting heavy pans and dishes out of the dishwasher may cause discomfort.

✓ Help out with the laundry. Carry filled laundry baskets up and down the stairs. If you hang clothes outside to dry, carry wet laundry to the clothesline. When the laundry basket is filled, offer to carry it to wherever your partner wants to put it away. If you do your laundry at a laundromat, go along with her. Help her put dirty clothes in the washers and wet clothes in the dryers. Fold dry clothes together.

✓ Do any heavy lifting. Empty the trash in the house, and take the garbage cans out to the curb.

✓ Put away any items that require climbing, such as seldom-used dishes in high cabinets. If a light bulb needs to be changed in a ceiling fixture, take care of it.

✓ Purchase household cleaners that are environmentally safe and pregnant-woman-friendly. Some cleaners have strong odors that may make the mom-to-be feel ill. Others are not safe to use during pregnancy. Read product labels for information on toxicity.

✓ Take over chores that require long periods of standing, such as ironing or doing the dishes. If you don't want to iron, take items to the laundry or pay someone to iron them.

✓ Go shopping for food and other necessities when your partner is too fatigued to do it. Together make a list of what you need, then you can go to the store.

✓ Run errands when you can to allow your partner to rest. Plan a trip to take clothes to the dry cleaner, get gasoline, go to the drugstore and make other stops.

✓ Share the cooking, especially if your partner experiences nausea and vomiting. In some cases, it may be the only food you'll get!

Some women find that cooking odors make them feel very ill, and cooking is the last thing they want to do.

✓ Be sure her car is in good working order. Check the tire pressure, be sure oil levels, water levels and other fluid levels are full, keep it filled with gas and keep it clean.

Making Your Home and Her Environment Safe

There are a lot of things you can do to make your environment safe for the mom-to-be. Keeping your home safe is one way you can ensure your growing baby is not exposed to situations that could harm it. Steps you take now can help your partner avoid accidents and reduce the risk of exposure to harmful substances. All it takes is a little planning and foresight.

EMPTY THE KITTY LITTER. Even if the cat is your partner's or you are not particularly fond of it, empty the litter box to reduce the mom-to-be's exposure to toxoplasmosis. *Toxoplasmosis* is a disease spread by contact with an infected cat or its feces. Your partner can pick up the protozoa from the cat's litter box, from surfaces the cat walks on or from the cat itself when she pets it. Keep cats off counters and tables. Suggest your partner wash her hands thoroughly after every contact with the cat, and advise her not to nuzzle it or to kiss it.

The disease can also be contracted from eating infected raw meat, drinking infected raw goat's milk, eating infected raw eggs or eating food contaminated by insects. To prevent transmission of the microorganism, cook foods thoroughly, use hygienic measures in the kitchen and avoid eating any food that could be contaminated. Infection in the mother-to-be during pregnancy can lead to miscarriage or an infected infant at birth.

HELP AVOID EXPOSURE TO DISEASES. It's important for your partner to avoid exposure to various diseases when possible. This includes chicken pox, measles and mumps, if she's never been exposed to any of them. Other diseases can cause problems, such as fifth disease, also called *parvovirus 19*, hepatitis, gastrointestinal problems and Lyme disease. Avoid situations in which your partner could be exposed. If you know there's an outbreak of fifth disease (most likely in daycare situations and schools), advise her to be careful and to avoid exposure. Try to choose places to eat that are clean and practice good sanitation. Don't go hiking in an area full of ticks that carry Lyme disease.

MAINTAINING BODY TEMPERATURE.   An elevated body temperature in a pregnant woman for an extended period may harm her growing baby. For this reason, your partner should avoid environments that can raise her body temperature, such as soaking in hot tubs, saunas and spas. Steam rooms should also be avoided.

In addition, there is some controversy about the safety of using electric blankets during pregnancy. Until we know more, stay warm using other methods, such as putting a down comforter or extra blankets on the bed. Or snuggle together to stay warm. Avoid using an electric blanket or electric mattress pad.

Some Precautions for Environmental Poisons

You should be aware of how the environment can affect your partner's health and that of the developing baby. There are many environmental poisons and pollutants that can harm a developing fetus; they include lead, mercury and pesticides.

Lead is readily transported across the placenta to the baby; toxicity can occur as early as the 12th week of pregnancy. Exposure to lead increases the chance of miscarriage. Lead exposure can come from many sources, including water pipes, solders, storage batteries, some construction materials, paints, dyes and wood preservatives. Try to ensure that your partner is not exposed to lead by keeping your home free of these substances.

IN THE DOGHOUSE

Don't put off doing something to make your home or your partner's environment safe. Her safety means safety for your growing baby.

Exposure to *mercury* occurs when someone eats contaminated fish; one report linked contaminated grain to mercury poisoning. Reports link exposure of a mother-to-be to cerebral palsy and microcephaly in the fetus.

Make sure any fish you eat is not contaminated, and try to keep consumption of fish to no more than 12 ounces a week.

Pesticide exposure is common because of the extensive use of pesticides to control unwanted plant growth; those of most concern include DDT, chlordane, heptachlor and lindane. Exposure to pesticides during pregnancy may increase the rate of miscarriage and fetal-growth restriction. Stop using pesticides in your home during pregnancy to avoid the mom-to-be's exposure.

You may not be able to eliminate all contact with pesticides. To protect your partner and yourself against them, avoid exposure when possible. Thoroughly wash all fruits and vegetables before eating them. If you know you will be around certain chemicals, wash your hands thoroughly after exposure. Don't let your partner handle any of the substances listed above, and try to avoid exposing her to any of them.

You may also bring substances into your home on your work clothes. If you think you may be exposing the mom-to-be to hazardous substances in this manner, be sure to discuss it with your partner and the doctor at one of the first prenatal visits.

Safety Tips for around the House

There are some things you can do to help increase safety in your home. These ideas are fairly simple to implement and don't cost a lot of money or take a lot of time. But they're well worth it if one of them prevents an accident!

✓ Use a nonskid mat or special appliqués on the floor of the tub or shower to prevent slips or falls. This becomes more important as pregnancy progresses because your partner's center of gravity shifts, and her balance may be affected. If you have old mats or appliqués, think about replacing them now.

✓ Outside the tub or shower, be sure bath mats are skid-free. If the backing is starting to fall off, replace the mat.

✓ Use night lights in your home or leave a lamp on at night so your partner doesn't trip over something in the dark if she gets up to go to the bathroom (and she probably will).

✓ Be sure outside walk areas and paths that she uses are well lit.

✓ When it snows, shovel sidewalks and paths so it's easy for your partner to walk on them. Try to keep ice accumulation down to avoid places where the mom-to-be could slip and fall.

✓ Put away all cleaning supplies that contain toxic chemicals. Buy environmentally friendly products for use during pregnancy.

✓ If you're going to paint the baby's room before birth, do it yourself. A pregnant woman should avoid exposure to paint fumes. Open all the windows to keep fresh air coming in when you paint.

✓ Be sure the fish you eat is not contaminated. Check Chapter 2 for a list of fish to avoid.

✓ Thoroughly wash all fruits and vegetables before eating to remove any pesticides and other contaminants.

✓ Wash your hands thoroughly after each trip to the bathroom, after you have come in contact with raw meat or poultry or after petting an animal.

✓ Check out your small appliances to be sure they are in good working order and the cords are OK.

✓ Encourage your partner to follow directions provided with your microwave oven for safe use during pregnancy.

Seat Belt and Shoulder Harness Use during Pregnancy

Should your partner wear her seat belt and shoulder harness during pregnancy? Yes! These safety restraints are just as necessary during pregnancy as before or after pregnancy.

For her protection and the protection of your developing baby, your partner should *always wear her safety belt when driving or riding in a vehicle!* There is no evidence that use of safety restraints increases the chance of fetal or uterine injury. Both your partner and baby have a better chance of survival in an accident if she wears her seat belt.

There is a correct way to wear a safety belt during pregnancy. Your partner should place the lap-belt part of the restraint under her abdomen and across her upper thighs so it's snug but comfortable. Next, she should adjust the sitting position so the belt crosses her shoulder without cutting into her neck. The shoulder harness should be positioned between her breasts, not slipped off her shoulder. The lap belt cannot hold her safely by itself, especially during pregnancy.

4

Changes in Your Life as the Expectant Dad

Many of the changes your partner experiences during pregnancy will affect you in a lot of ways, if they haven't already. There have been, and will continue to be, numerous adjustments in your life during this pregnancy. Pregnancy definitely affects you!

During this pregnancy, you may be doing more around the house because you want to help out or because your partner is unable to do much. You may be doing more cooking or cleaning now. You may be going to prenatal appointments or taking your partner to various prenatal tests. You may have curtailed your work schedule, or you may be traveling less. Whatever changes you've made, you probably made them because of the effect they have on your life with your partner and your desire to be an active participant in the pregnancy.

You may be looking to your future by talking about baby names with the mom-to-be, discussing if your partner should continue working or whether you will be a stay-at-home dad. If you both plan to return to work, you may want to discuss what type of child-care arrangements you intend to check out. You may be concerned

---

Chapter Focus

As a father-to-be, during pregnancy you may have to make some changes in how often you participate in various activities or when you do them. This chapter covers some changes you may need to make in your life as your partner's pregnancy progresses—including changes at work, social changes, travel (your individual travel and travel as a couple), your participation in various activities during the pregnancy, such as sports, hunting, fishing or "going out with the guys"—and laws that can help you during the pregnancy and after baby's birth.

We also provide information if you are an older dad or if you are an unmarried partner. Both of these situations may create unique conditions.

Our goal is to help you understand what changes you may need to make, to realize why they are necessary and to provide you with some guidelines on ways to make life happy and satisfying for you and your partner.

about your financial situation or making plans for your family's financial future. (This is covered in depth in Chapter 7.)

As you have probably learned by now, you are involved in the pregnancy. And your involvement demonstrates to your partner that your growing baby is important to you, too.

It's important to continue to be involved in the pregnancy as much as you are willing and able to be. Dealing with the changes that may occur—for you and your partner—in the coming months can help make this involvement more meaningful to you.

COMMON FEELINGS YOU MAY EXPERIENCE

You may feel many emotions as pregnancy progresses—excitement about becoming a dad, increased anxiety about what lies ahead, concern about changes in your couple relationship, thrill at the thought of finally becoming a family. You may not have many worries at all and feel totally happy about the pregnancy. Some feelings experienced by a father-to-be include:

✓ feeling somewhat ignored because attention is focused on your partner and the growing baby

✓ feeling elated about the thought of becoming a dad

✓ being a little jealous and "feeling left out"

✓ being anxious about the impending labor and delivery

✓ worrying about the mom-to-be's health and that of the growing baby

✓ thinking about all the wonderful things you'll do with your child in the years to come

✓ helping your partner deal with the pain of childbirth

✓ concern over changes in your sex life

✓ being thrilled about your partner's pregnancy

✓ anxiety about whether you will be a good dad

✓ nervousness about being able to handle a baby or dropping the baby

✓ wondering how your finances are going to be affected by the birth and new baby

✓ making sure you have enough time for baby

✓ fear that relatives will visit too often

✓ concern about losing the relationship with your partner after baby's birth

✓ loss of personal freedom

✓ providing adequately for the family

✓ dealing with baby's crying

These are all normal feelings. Don't be disturbed or feel you are unusual if you experience any of them. Realize they are all part of being an expectant dad. Just relax; you don't need to master every-thing in the first few weeks of the pregnancy or soon after baby's birth. Take your time, and learn what's right for you and your new family.

BROWNIE POINTS

Discussing any fears you have about being a good father helps your partner realize how involved you are in the pregnancy. It also allows her to help you overcome those fears by addressing them together.

Are You Experiencing Morning Sickness?

Some expectant fathers experience various physical problems during a partner's pregnancy; it is called *couvade*. The term comes from a Carib Indian tribe in which all fathers-to-be participate in rituals that enable a man to understand a little more what his pregnant partner is experiencing. In our culture, a father-to-be may experience nausea, headache, back and muscle aches, insomnia, fatigue or depression. These can be very real physical discomforts, so if you have any of them, it may not be "all in your head."

CHANGES YOU MAY NEED OR WANT TO MAKE IN YOUR LIFE

Changes in Your Work Situation

Are you a busy professional who puts in long hours at work or on the job? Do you travel out of town a great deal? Are you forced to be away from home a lot? If any of these situations applies to you, you may want to think about making some changes. Why? There are several reasons—to give yourself some time to enjoy your life with your partner before your baby arrives, to be available to help out at home with chores and tasks, to prepare for baby's arrival and to take care of your partner if she has problems.

One change you might consider making is to cut down on travel, especially as your partner's due date approaches. No one, not even a doctor who's had a lot of experience delivering babies, can accurately predict when a woman will go into labor. If you are away on a business trip, you may miss your baby's birth. If your partner experiences any problems during pregnancy, you may have to help out at home or take care of her, so this may limit travel.

If you work long hours, you may want to make changes so you can be home more often. If your job includes shift work, you may ask about changing your schedule. When possible, discuss working from home with your employer. This may be an option you haven't explored in the past.

Examine your job situation, and investigate ways you can make changes that are beneficial for all of you. Discuss any changes with your partner and your employer.

Changes in Your Social Life

You may be wondering what kind of changes you might have to make in your social lives. A few situations could impact on your partner's health and her quality of life. Some areas that may need to be addressed include the following.

✓ Don't stay out late at night—if the mom-to-be tires easily, being a night owl may take its toll on her. If she needs a lot of rest, be considerate and go home early.

✓ Avoid places where people smoke a lot—spending a great deal of time in bars or nightclubs isn't a good idea because of the secondary smoke, which can affect a pregnant woman and her developing baby.

✓ Forego activities in which your pregnant partner is exposed to loud noises—concerts and other events where the fetus may be bombarded with extremely loud noises aren't good for baby's developing hearing. It can also be very fatiguing for a woman to be exposed to excessive noise for an extended period of time.

✓ Reconsider eating out—this can be a problem for a woman who experiences nausea and vomiting; food may be one of the last things she wants to have to deal with. If weight gain is a concern, you may want to avoid restaurant food because of the portion sizes and the richness of the food. You don't have to give up eating out completely, but you may want to save the experience for special occasions. You both may feel more comfortable eating most of your meals at home. You can help out by offering to do a lot of the cooking, if you aren't already.

✓ Ask your partner whether she wants to accompany you to various activities—a pregnant woman may feel very uncomfortable sitting in the bleachers while you play softball or camping out in a beach chair watching you play rugby. Let her make the decision as to whether she wants to put her comfort on hold.

It's not unusual to have to adapt your life to the comfort of your pregnant partner. These are ways to show you are considerate of how the mom-to-be is coping with a growing pregnancy. These changes are only the first steps in the many you will probably have to make after baby arrives!

Changes in Travel Activities

TRAVELING FOR YOUR JOB. In your professional capacity, you may be required to do a little or a lot of traveling. If so, it may be impossible to cut travel completely out of your job, but you may want to think about making some changes in how

IN THE DOGHOUSE

Don't make travel plans for yourself during the last 6 weeks of the pregnancy. If you do go out of town, you may miss your baby's birth.

often you travel, how far you go and how long you are gone. This may be especially true if your partner suffers from any problems during pregnancy that necessitate your being there, such as if she is confined to bed.

Toward the end of the pregnancy, medical situations may occur that would make you want to be there, such as pre-eclampsia or placenta previa. If your company requires you to travel, try to limit the amount of time you are away from home, especially during the last 6 weeks.

> ## BROWNIE POINTS
>
> Asking your partner about participating in an activity before you make a commitment is courteous and lets her know you're thinking about her feelings.

After examining your travel requirements, if you believe you can make any changes to your travel schedule, discuss it as soon as possible with your employer. Explain the situation, and see if compromises can be reached.

TRAVELING AS A COUPLE.   Traveling during pregnancy for a pregnant woman can be tiring and frustrating, but if pregnancy is normal, your partner should be able to travel in the first and second trimesters without too much trouble. The best time to travel is during the second trimester. Your partner should talk to the doctor if she is considering travel in the third trimester.

Pregnancy does impose some restrictions and limitations on traveling. If you travel together, your partner's discomfort level is likely to increase, especially if she is cooped up in a car or on a plane for hours. She may have trouble sleeping in a strange bed. If the mom-to-be develops a complication while you're away from home, it may be difficult to find good care. Medical personnel who have been involved in the pregnancy and know her history will not be available to care for her. Some doctors won't accept a pregnant woman as a patient because they don't know her medical history.

If there have been complications during pregnancy, avoid travel as much as possible. Don't plan on traveling during the last 6 weeks. Labor could begin at any time, her bag of waters could break or other problems could occur. The doctor who has treated her during the pregnancy knows her and has a record of tests she's had, which is important information. It doesn't make sense to take chances.

Many women want to know if the doctor can tell when they will go into labor so they can travel. Unfortunately, no one can predict when labor will begin. Always discuss any travel plans with your partner and the doctor before you finalize them (in other words, before you buy nonrefundable tickets!).

Changes in Your Personal Activities

Do you play a lot of sports? Do you go on fishing or hunting trips fairly often? Do you go out with the guys on a fairly regular basis? You may want, or you may find it necessary, to curtail some of these activities during the pregnancy. A pregnant woman needs and welcomes the support of her partner.

Your life is in the process of changing now. After your baby's birth, you will no longer be just a couple. Very soon, you will be a family, and being a good parent requires your time and commitment to the task. Begin to focus on ways you can help each other. Accept the responsibility of being a father now.

We are not suggesting you give up all your free time or stop all your activities and stay at home. How-

IN THE DOGHOUSE

Don't ignore the impact your partner's pregnancy may have on your social, sports or "guy" activities. She needs your support during this time, so be willing to give up some things you might normally do.

ever, we are pointing out that some adjustments may have to be made in the choices you make. Discuss your plans with your partner; ask her what changes she would like you to make. Make changes together. By working together, you can reach a balance that satisfies your needs and those of the mom-to-be.

LAWS YOU SHOULD KNOW ABOUT

In the last few years, Congress has passed various laws to protect pregnant women who wanted to work during their pregnancies. In the past, women were not encouraged to work—in fact, many were prevented from working while they were pregnant, even if they didn't have any problems and felt OK. A positive result of the passage of these laws is that many of them also affect men. Unfortunately, few men take advantage of them. Various laws, and how they can affect you, are discussed below.

The Pregnancy Discrimination Act

The Pregnancy Discrimination Act of 1978 requires companies employing 15 or more people to treat pregnant workers the same way they treat other workers who have medical disabilities and cannot work. The law prohibits job discrimination on the basis of pregnancy, childbirth or related disability. It guarantees equal treatment of all disabilities, including pregnancy, birth or related medical conditions. Although this law does not directly affect you, it is important to know about it, in case your partner encounters any problems at her place of work due to pregnancy-related complications.

Maternity Leave

Maternity leave is the period during which a woman's physician states she cannot work after delivery of her baby. This can range from 4 to 6 weeks after a vaginal birth to 6 to 8 weeks following a Cesarean delivery. Fathers are not covered under this law.

The Family and Medical Leave Act

The Family and Medical Leave Act was passed in 1993, and it covers women and men. This law gives millions of fathers the same right to spend time with their baby in the first year of life as women have been granted.

If you have worked for your present employer for at least 1 year, the law allows a new parent (man or woman) to take up to 12 weeks of unpaid leave in any 12-month period for the birth of a baby. To be eligible, you must work at your job for at least 1,250 hours a year (about 60% of a normal 40-hour work week). In addition, if both parents work for the same employer, only a *total* of 12 weeks off between them is allowed. This act applies only to companies that employ 50 or more people within a 75-mile radius. States may allow an employer to deny job restoration to employees in the top 10% compensation bracket.

Any time taken off before the birth of a baby is counted toward the 12 weeks a person is entitled to in any given year. (Taking time before the birth might be necessary in a situation in which a woman needs her partner's help because she is having health/medical problems.) Leave may be taken intermittently or all at the same time.

Consider taking advantage of this law. You will soon learn how quickly babies grow and change. This is an excellent opportunity to be a part of an incredible time in the life of your child.

If you are covered under this law, you must be restored to an equivalent position with equal benefits when you return to your job. If you have any questions, check with your state's labor office. For further information on the Family and Medical Leave Act, you can also call their hot line at 800-522-0925.

State Laws

Many states have passed legislation that deals with parental leave. Laws differ, so check with your state's labor office, or consult the personnel director in your company's human resources department if you have questions.

If You Want to Take Leave . . .

Even though laws have been passed to safeguard your right to take paternity leave, the fact is most men don't. If you decide this is something you want to do, you may be a trailblazer in your company in this area, so you may have to make an extra effort to be granted your rights.

How Many Men Take Paternity Leave?

Although men have been granted the right, under certain circumstances, to take paternity leave to stay home with a new baby, most men don't take advantage of it. Only about 20% of all new fathers take any time off, and they use only 1 or 2 weeks of leave.

One survey reported that those interviewed believed they couldn't afford to take time off (because of the lack of income while they were on leave), or they were afraid they would jeopardize their careers if they took a leave of absence to stay at home with a new baby.

Fathers who have done it in the past offer some suggestions about how to approach the subject with your employer and outline steps you may have to take. Consider the following actions.

✓ *Know your rights under the law.* If you and your employer meet the criteria described above, you are guaranteed paternity-leave rights under the Family and Medical Leave Act. It may be necessary to educate your employer about this law, if others in the company have not taken advantage of it. Don't be put off by an employer who claims you can't take leave from your job. Get the facts, and present them to your employer.

✓ *Be prepared to negotiate.* You may decide you want to take 12 full weeks off after your partner returns to her job. Your employer may not be able to let you go for that length of time. You'll have to work it out to the satisfaction of you both so you each get what you want. In a situation such as the one described here, you might instead ask for 6 weeks off at one time, then two 3-week periods later.

✓ *Be willing to compromise.* You may want to spend your time at home, free from the pressures of your job so you can concentrate on your new baby. Your employer may want you to be involved in your job, even if you're not at the company offices. If there is some give-and-take to your negotiations, you may each come out a winner. You might consider taking phone calls or doing paperwork from home a few days a week. Or you might be able to work on your home computer during the day or when your partner is home and can tend the baby. If you and your employer are willing to consider creative solutions, you may both get what you want.

✓ *It's important to be persistent.* This may be a new situation or an unusual request for your employer, so don't give up if you don't get what you want the first time. Your employer may have to check out your state laws or may need information from the federal government on what the Family and Medical Leave Act is and how it protects you.

✓ *If leave is important to you, check on it (or negotiate for it) at your next job.* If you believe this may be important to you in the future, ask about paternity leave when interviewing for any new position. You may be pleasantly surprised by how a company responds to requests for leave after a baby's birth.

WILL YOU BE AN OLDER DAD?

Having a baby at any age is a big decision.

Today, it's not uncommon for an older man to father a child. Some men choose to wait until their careers are established to get married and become a father. Others may be in a second marriage to a woman who wants children. Still others have older, grown children and decide to begin another family with their partner. Whatever the situation, many older men are finding themselves expectant dads.

Being older when you become a parent can have some very positive benefits. One positive aspect of this situation is that an older man may have more time and patience to be a father. Many young fathers find it difficult to spend a lot of time with their young children because of career responsibilities and travel commitments. There are other pluses—an older father usually exhibits greater self-confidence. Older fathers may also be more financially secure; the fact that an older dad may be established in his career is an added bonus. Older men may be more willing and able to spend quality time with their children, doing many different types of activities. And studies have shown that as men get older, they become more nurturing and supportive, and are often more affectionate with a child than a younger man might be.

Some of the less-positive aspects of being an older dad include the fact that some older men may have physical limitations. They may

---

**MEMORABLE MOMENTS
FROM DR. DAD**

At Marnie's 6-week postpartum checkup, she was doing well. She seemed to be in good spirits and looking forward to returning to work in another 6 weeks. She told me that her husband had decided to take off 6 weeks from his teaching job to stay home to take care of their son, Tom, when she returned to work.

When I next saw Marnie, I asked her how things had gone for her husband during his paternity leave. She told me it had been an incredible bonding experience for him and the baby. He felt very confident in being able to care for Tom on his own, and he had a better appreciation for what is required of a parent. It was a positive experience for all of them.

not have as much energy for robust activities or physical play interactions. Fathers who are over 55 may fear not seeing their child get married or have children of his or her own.

An older man must be sure he is physically and mentally prepared to deal with the demands of fatherhood. He must have some supply of energy to deal with raising a child.

No matter what age a father-to-be is, it's good to keep in mind what really makes a good father. The most important elements of being a good parent include spending quality time with the child, responding to his or her needs, providing security and being involved in a child's life. If you are willing to commit to these goals, parenting at any age will be rewarding.

Some Challenges for You

Pregnancy for an older man may be more challenging than it is for someone younger. You may find it more difficult or demanding keeping up with the changes that are occurring in your life.

If this is the case in your situation, discuss it with your partner. Explain what you are willing and able to do. Ask her to be specific in her requests for your help. Tell her you will give of your time to help her out. Because you are probably more nurturing and caring, you may be emotionally more supportive of her and the experiences she is undergoing.

ARE YOU AN UNMARRIED EXPECTANT FATHER?

Some couples today choose to have a child without being married; situations vary from couple to couple. This situation can raise many issues for a couple. Being part of that couple can raise particular issues for you.

In this section, we attempt to provide questions for you to consider and to think about; we offer no answers. These questions are of a legal nature that we are not qualified to answer. However, we have included them here because your role as a father may have legal ramifications. You may want to consider using the questions we have listed below as a basis for formulating questions about your own situation to discuss with an attorney, a patient advocate, a hospital social worker or someone else qualified to give you answers.

Some questions you may want to think about and to discuss with someone knowledgeable about the situation include those listed below. After reading these questions, you may have others that you wish to address. To learn what applies to you in your particular case, we suggest you contact a specialist in family law in your area.

> ## My Mother-in-Law Said
>
> *If a pregnant woman eats sour foods, her baby will have a sour disposition.*
>
> Some aspects of your baby's personality are set while it is developing in the womb. Other aspects develop from exposure to the environment and parenting styles after he or she is born. The foods a pregnant woman eats have no effect on whether baby is happy or difficult.

✓ My partner and I aren't married, and I don't know if we ever will be. How does this situation affect me as my baby's father?

✓ What if we decide to get married in the future—how may what we do now affect that?

✓ What are my legal rights if we never get married?

✓ If we go our separate ways later, can I have equal custody of my child?

✓ Do we need to set up a legal guardianship for our baby, in case something happens to both of us?

✓ Do my parents have legal rights in regard to their grandchild (my child)?

✓ I've heard that in some states, my name may not be on the baby's birth certificate. Is that true?

✓ Can I be involved in making medical decisions for my partner and my expected baby during the labor and delivery, or after the birth?

✓ If anything happens to my partner, can I make medical decisions for our baby after it is born?

✓ What type of arrangements must I make for my child in case of my partner's death?

✓ What kind of arrangements can I make in my will to ensure my child will be taken care of in the event of my death?

✓ Do I need to name a guardian in my will for my child in case of my death and my partner's death at the same time?

5

Your Couple
Relationship

Your relationship as a couple undergoes many changes during pregnancy. If you work at it, these changes can be positive. Some occur because your roles are different now. Others happen when a couple's emotions come into play. You may both feel stressed by what you are experiencing. If this is your first pregnancy, the newness and unpredictability of it all may seem overwhelming at times.

The best advice we can give you is to *work together* to maintain your closeness. Be considerate of each other, and support one another physically and emotionally. Although you will no longer be only a "couple" after your baby is born—you'll be a family—your interactions with your partner and her interactions with you are still very important. In the months after your baby's birth, you'll depend on each other a great deal as you begin the challenges of parenting.

Whatever you do, don't ignore your relationship now or after baby is born. Don't let courtesy and caring slip away. Strive to maintain the bond that brought you to this point in your lives. Make it a labor of love.

Chapter Focus

In this chapter, we attempt to help you preserve and increase the passion and devotion you have for each other as a couple. We explore how emotions (yours and your partner's) may be affected by pregnancy. We investigate what is normal during this time, so you won't feel like you're the only person who's ever experienced these feelings. We discuss sex, which can be very important to you both during pregnancy. We look at issues that promote intimacy for a couple. We also examine massage techniques you may want to try to help make your partner feel better. And lastly, we look into ways you can bond with your unborn baby.

DO YOU FEEL LIKE YOU'RE ON AN EMOTIONAL ROLLER COASTER?

During pregnancy, your partner's physical changes often contribute to her emotional feelings. And her feelings will probably affect you.

Although men usually present a strong front emotionally, many are affected by pregnancy.

Some Common Feelings Men Have

You may experience many emotions during this pregnancy. You may feel anxious about your ability to be a good father or to provide for your new family. You may be worried that sex with your partner might harm the baby. You may feel removed or a little jealous. You may be questioning how this new person in your lives will affect your couple relationship. These are concerns men commonly express.

Set aside some quiet time together, and talk to your partner about your feelings. You might be surprised to learn she has the same concerns. Be open and direct—it can help you both. Be actively involved in the pregnancy, such as going to prenatal visits, reading books and articles to learn more about pregnancy, birth and the new baby, and participating in childbirth-education classes. If you have a better understanding of what may occur in pregnancy, you may feel more confident about handling what comes along. Try to view your pregnancy as an opportunity to grow closer. It can be a time for your relationship to become deeper and more meaningful as you work together through the pregnancy and prepare for baby.

As pregnancy progresses, you may become a little more anxious. This increased anxiety may be caused by your concerns about your partner's health, the health of the baby, labor and delivery, and your ability to be a good dad.

There are some things you can do to reassure your partner and yourself. They may help you grow more comfortable with handling the ups and downs of pregnancy and help you accept your role of father. Consider the following suggestions, and use what works for you.

✓ Tell your partner what level of participation you are comfortable with in the baby's birth. Discuss what she expects of you.

✓ Let your partner know it helps you when she acknowledges your assistance. You may be more willing to offer to help if you know it means something to the mom-to-be.

✓ Find out what you can do for your partner during pregnancy to make her life, and yours, a little easier. Ask for suggestions. These might include such things as keeping stress to a minimum, being patient, promoting good nutrition and exercise, helping around the house, planning for the baby's arrival, and reading, studying and preparing together.

✓ Ask your partner to listen to you when you talk. Express your hopes, fears and expectations about the baby's birth and being a good father. This may be a little difficult at first, but it's worth the effort.

✓ Discuss how you will divide responsibilities now and after the baby comes. List what you can do and what your partner can do. If possible, practice before baby's birth!

Early Pregnancy

In early pregnancy, physical adjustments and changes can take their toll on the mom-to-be. Fatigue, frequent urination, and nausea and vomiting can make life fairly uncomfortable for her. She may respond in various ways. She may be so tired that all she can do is rest and sleep, leaving you to fend for yourself. She may be so sick with nausea and vomiting that the thought of going near the kitchen sends her running for the bathroom. Her moods may be unpredictable, and she may cry over every little thing. An innocent comment from you may send her into a tizzy. These changes are common and a natural part of pregnancy—knowing that may help you deal with them without becoming emotional yourself.

BROWNIE POINTS

Keep a positive attitude, and pass it along to your pregnant partner! Studies show that when a couple is optimistic about pregnancy, labor and delivery, the outcome is far better than for those couples who are pessimistic.

One way to help your partner during these rough times is to focus on a healthy lifestyle. Eat nutritious foods together (when she can eat), and exercise as a couple, even if it's just a walk around the

IN THE DOGHOUSE

If you find your partner is more emotionally dependent on you now, accept it. Many women feel more dependent on their partners during pregnancy because of the many challenges they face. If the mom-to-be has been independent in the past, and she now depends on you more for all sorts of things, realize it is probably due to the pregnancy.

block. Allow your partner to rest when she needs it. If either of you smoke, make an effort to give it up now, and avoid alcohol or drugs.

Try to maintain your cool. Keep in mind that being emotional is a common symptom of pregnancy and is caused by your partner's changing hormones. If you understand that these hormonal changes are normal and necessary for a healthy pregnancy—they're for the good of your developing baby—it may help you deal with situations without getting angry or upset.

The Second Trimester

The middle part of pregnancy is usually the best time for everyone. Hormonal changes have settled down and are not quite so dramatic. Nausea and vomiting are often gone, your partner's body is adapting to the changes and the baby hasn't grown large enough to cause her discomfort. Energy levels may become more normal, and your partner may feel pretty good. She may seem more like her prepregnancy self!

It is during this time that movement of the baby begins to be felt, and the fetus often becomes more real to you both. As the mom-to-be's abdomen grows and her pregnancy becomes more obvious, becoming a parent in the near future isn't so hard to imagine now. Your partner may have an ultrasound, during which you may see a moving picture of your baby—you may even find out if it's a girl or a boy!

You may be more emotional during this time; don't be surprised if it happens. As the baby becomes more real to you, you may feel overwhelmed at the thought of what lies ahead. You may have many of the common anxieties as other dads-to-be. It's OK—it just means you're normal.

Continue to take good care of your partner, and take good care of yourself, too. Eat well, and get enough rest. Exercise can help relieve stress. Talk about your feelings with your partner; let her know what you're thinking and planning. It can also help to talk to other men in your situation—both expectant fathers and men who already have children. It helps relieve your anxiety to know you aren't the only man who has ever felt the way you feel now.

Your Baby Is Coming Soon

In the last part of pregnancy, you will see great changes in your partner's body. These changes are caused by the baby's rapid growth, which can cause discomfort for your partner. She may have to go to the bathroom a lot again, and she may have trouble sleeping. She may not want to do too much because it's hard to get around, and the growing baby may be encroaching upon her lung space, making any exertions harder to deal with because she's not breathing as easily now.

You and your partner may be anxious to get the pregnancy over with. At the same time, she may be a little fearful about how well she will handle labor and delivery. She may also be wondering how you will handle it all and whether the birth experience will change how you feel about her.

Be supportive of your partner. Do as much as you can around the house—tend to chores, fix meals and run errands when the mom-to-be doesn't have the time or energy to do them. Your partner may need you to be her cheerleader right now—you may need to bolster her confidence that she will do a good job and that you can get through this together. At the same time, encourage her to be active and to do what she can. She'll feel a lot better "doing something" than just sitting around.

Help yourself by attending childbirth-education classes together so you'll both be prepared for baby's arrival. Let your partner know how much you are willing to be involved in labor and delivery.

Attend as many prenatal appointments with her as you can, especially during the last part of the pregnancy. You and your partner can discuss with the doctor what might happen and ways to deal with various situations. You'll have a better understanding of what lies ahead and how you can help each other through this incredible experience.

Don't make unrealistic demands on the mom-to-be. It's not unusual to hear a woman say she's not going to use medication for pain relief during labor or delivery because "my partner doesn't want me to." Let her make those important decisions, based on what she knows about herself and how she handles pain. Get behind her in whatever she chooses, but let her know these important decisions are hers to make.

The end of the pregnancy will be upon you soon, and the emotions you are feeling now will change. However, they will be replaced by other, different emotions as you take on the role of "dad."

SEXUAL INTIMACY—IS IT OK?

Sex. It's an important part of any couple's relationship. After all, it's how you got here in the first place, isn't it?

You may be a little anxious about sexual activity during pregnancy—a man is more often concerned with this aspect of a couple's relationship than the woman is. However, you don't need to worry about it too much. Most doctors agree sex can be a part of a normal, low-risk pregnancy. But because it's important, and because you want to be reassured it's OK in your situation, you and your partner should discuss it with the doctor at a prenatal visit.

Normal sexual activity doesn't harm a growing baby. Neither intercourse nor orgasm should be a problem with a normal, low-risk pregnancy. A baby is well protected inside the uterus by the amniotic sac and amniotic fluid. Uterine muscles are strong and protect the baby. A thick mucus plug seals the cervix, which also offers protection.

As a couple, you can usually continue the level of sexual activity you are used to. Frequent sexual activity should be OK, if that's what you both want. But keep in mind that sex doesn't just mean sexual intercourse. There are many ways for you to be sensual together, including giving each other a massage (see page 99), bathing together and talking about sex. Whatever you do, keep your sense of humor!

How Pregnancy May Affect a Woman's Sex Drive

A woman's sex-drive patterns can be different at different times during pregnancy, and they can also vary from the woman's normal pattern before

> ### Can Sex Start Labor?
>
> In the past, some researchers believed that if a couple had sex during the last few weeks of pregnancy, it might cause labor to start if the woman had an orgasm. (Orgasms release the hormone oxytocin; oxytocin can start contractions.) However, other researchers disagree. Because there is controversy about this situation, you and your partner should talk to the doctor about it at a prenatal visit. He or she will know what's best in your particular situation.

pregnancy. Women generally have one of two sex-drive patterns during pregnancy. The first is a lessening of desire in the first and third trimesters, with an increase in the second trimester. You may be surprised by the level of passion your partner exhibits. The second is a gradual decrease in desire for sex as pregnancy progresses.

Pregnancy may enhance the sex drive in some women. A woman may experience orgasms or multiple orgasms for the first time when she is pregnant. This is due to heightened hormonal activity and increased blood flow to the pelvic area. Your partner may also feel more voluptuous now, which can make her feel sexier.

You may find it necessary to explore new positions for lovemaking as pregnancy progresses. Your partner's growing abdomen may make some positions more uncomfortable for her than others. In addition, physicians advise a pregnant woman not to lie flat on her back after 16 weeks until the baby's birth because the weight of the uterus can restrict her circulation. Some couples find that experimenting during pregnancy leads to changes they continue to enjoy after the pregnancy is over.

How Sex during Pregnancy May Affect You

You may be a little surprised by how your partner's pregnancy affects you sexually. Men have expressed various feelings about having sex during pregnancy. The most common feelings are listed below.

✓ Fear you'll hurt the baby. You don't have to avoid sex for this reason. As discussed above and reiterated below, neither intercourse nor orgasm will hurt your baby.

✓ The baby is in the way, mentally *and* physically. Sometimes knowing your partner is pregnant can lessen your enthusiasm. Try to forget about it; instead concentrate on the pleasures you give and receive during sexual intimacy.

✓ Some men find it difficult to separate *maternal* and *sexy.* You may find yourself rethinking the way you look at your passionate partner of the past. Now she's a mother-to-be; do you have to treat her differently? Reflect on this if you feel this way. Your partner really hasn't changed; you don't have to change, either.

✓ You feel left out. As we've discussed, much of the attention is focused on your partner and the growing baby. But don't feel like you're not part of the action. You are a *very* important part, and the mom-to-be wouldn't be in this condition without you. Try to forget, or at least overlook, this aspect of the pregnancy, if it makes you a little uncomfortable.

✓ You may find your pregnant partner the most beautiful woman in the world. If so, tell her! For many men, a woman's enlarging bust, curvaceous body and glowing skin awaken feelings they didn't know they had. You may feel the need to take care of your partner and growing baby, and you may feel a sense of pride in creating life. These feelings may combine to make sex during pregnancy as good as, or even better than, ever!

Sex Myths You Can Probably Ignore

As we've already pointed out, sex may play a larger or smaller part in your lives as a pregnant couple. If your partner experiences a heightened sexual drive during pregnancy, enjoy it. Don't let common myths destroy your pleasure. Things that you may have heard might cause harm to the baby, which you can probably ignore, include the following.

✓ *Sex will harm the mom-to-be.* If you are careful about how you treat your partner, you won't hurt her during sexual intimacy. (Not lying on top of her tummy is probably the best advice we can give you.) Now's the time to experiment with new positions and new techniques. If you're still unsure, ask your partner what feels good to her.

✓ *Sex will hurt the baby.* No, it won't. The baby is well protected inside the womb. There's not much you can do, as far as sexual activity, that will harm a developing fetus.

✓ *Avoid oral sex.* You don't have to avoid oral sex if you both enjoy it. As your partner's pregnancy grows, oral sex may be one of the easiest ways for both of you to receive pleasure.

✓ *Sex may cause my partner's labor to start.* Studies report that this belief is unfounded in a normal, low-risk pregnancy. If you have questions, discuss them at one of your partner's prenatal visits.

When Should We Avoid Sexual Activity?

Some situations may keep you from having sex during pregnancy. If your partner has a history of miscarriage, the doctor may caution against sexual intercourse and orgasm; however, no data actually link the two. Avoid sexual activity if your partner experiences placenta previa or a low-lying placenta, an incompetent cervix, premature labor, multiple fetuses, a ruptured bag of waters, pain with intercourse, unexplained vaginal bleeding or discharge or if either of you has an unhealed herpes lesion or you believe labor has begun.

Sexual Practices to Avoid

Some sexual practices *should* be avoided during pregnancy. Don't insert any object into your partner's vagina that could cause injury or infection. *Never* blow air into the vagina; it is dangerous because it can force a potentially fatal air bubble into a woman's bloodstream. (This can occur whether or not a woman is pregnant.) Nipple stimulation releases oxytocin, which can cause uterine contractions; your partner might want to discuss this practice with the doctor.

YOUR INTIMACY AS A COUPLE

Intimacy is the private, personal, romantic relationship you experience as a couple. It is fundamental to your coupleship and essential to the emotional health you share. During this time of increased demands on your time and energies, it's important to foster and to promote intimacy between you. It will strengthen your relationship together, and it will contribute to your strength as a new family. Pregnancy is an opportunity to increase your intimacy as a couple.

Create Some Memories

One way to strengthen the bond you share as a couple is to create memories of this wonderful time you are sharing. By creating memories, you'll be able to recall the special moments you experienced and remember some of the funny or humorous events that occurred, too. Ways you can create memories of this pregnancy include those listed below.

✓ Keep a photographic record of the pregnancy. Take pictures every week—shots from the side are good ones—of how the mom-to-be's tummy is growing. You'll both enjoy looking at them for years to come!

✓ Provide your partner with a pregnancy journal to record her thoughts and feelings, such as the one we have written titled *Your Pregnancy Journal Week by Week*. We have places to write down physical and emotional changes she experiences, information from prenatal appointments, how baby is growing and developing, and her feelings as pregnancy progresses. Be sure you add your thoughts, too.

✓ Gather together baby pictures of you and your partner. Put them in an album to which you can also add pictures of your baby as he or she grows.

✓ Together make a list of pregnancy "firsts"—the first time you heard the heartbeat, the first baby picture (usually an ultrasound), when your partner first felt baby kick, when you first felt baby moving.

✓ Make a scrapbook of newspaper and magazine articles that speak to important issues today. You might consider adding to it as baby gets older.

✓ Make a cast of your partner's pregnant abdomen. You can make a tummy cast with plaster rolls available from an art-supply store. Cover her tummy with a water-soluble lubricant, apply the wet paper and let dry. You can also buy a kit to do this; check out www.bellymask.com on the Internet.

✓ If a tummy cast isn't for you, create a silhouette of your partner's tummy. Tape a large blank piece of paper to the wall. Shine a light on your partner to create a shadow on the paper, then trace it for a great keepsake. You could even frame it and hang it on the wall!

✓ On a videotape or a cassette tape, record your thoughts and feelings. Or videotape the mom-to-be's growing tummy at particular intervals, such as the first day of each month. It's fun to look back on or listen to as the years pass.

Keep Communicating

Another way to maintain your intimate relationship is to talk together about what you, the expectant dad, are going through and how you feel about it. It's not usually hard to get a woman to talk about her feelings—it's one thing women do fairly easily. However, many men find it harder to discuss their feelings. Society expects you to be stoic and bear things without complaining. So talking

---

MEMORABLE MOMENTS FROM DR. DAD

Jerry and Trista came to a prenatal visit looking uncomfortable. It took a while to find out what was bothering them, but after a few gentle questions, I heard from them both. Jerry said he was feeling a little frightened about having sex because he thought it might hurt the baby. He thought it could be dangerous and didn't want to do anything to cause problems. Trista was frustrated because she felt good, her pregnancy was going well and she thought sex was OK. Because the pregnancy was uncomplicated and Trista was doing well, I reassured them that sex during pregnancy was safe. Jerry looked quite relieved, and they left the office with big smiles on both their faces.

about and discussing what's happening and how you feel may be something you haven't done much before. Now may be a good time to take a stab at it.

Try to open up communication between you and your partner, even if it's something you don't normally do. One good way to begin is to start a list of baby names. Get some books of baby names, and go through them together. As you discuss names, approach subjects that are a little harder to talk about, such as what your feelings are about becoming a dad or your expectations about your financial future. Or talk about what you want to do in the nursery. As you look at paint chips and wallpaper samples, you can begin discussing subjects that are harder for you to talk about.

Many men don't want to burden their partner with topics that might not interest her or issues they believe are irrelevant. However, most women welcome the chance to talk about these things. Some women may not be quite as interested as you are in finances, for example, but talking about them allows both of you to share your thoughts and plan together this very important aspect of your lives. And you may be pleasantly surprised, too, when the mom-to-be expresses more of an interest than you expected.

The important point is to make an effort to keep communications open between you. It will help your relationship, and it may be just what your partner needs right now. And it may also help you.

Relax Together
Relaxing together can help you regroup and re-energize for the challenges ahead. As strange as it may sound, you may have to work at relaxing, but you'll be glad you did. Your relaxation periods can give you a clearer focus on what is important to you as a couple.

There are many techniques you can use to help you relax. One way is to turn off the phones and find a quiet space to share. Keep the lights low; light some candles. Scented candles can provide dim light *and* aromatherapy at the same time. Play soft, soothing music. To help your partner relax, pay attention to your breathing; focus on it until you are both breathing easily and rhythmically. (This technique can be useful during labor.) Allow yourselves to drift off so you feel as if you are floating on clouds.

Other ways to relax include doing gentle stretches together. They can help your partner stay flexible and limber. Giving your partner a gentle, all-over body rub with a good moisturizer may also help keep her skin soft. Learn some meditation techniques—books in the library can be a good source. Practice them together.

MASSAGE TECHNIQUES TO RELIEVE PREGNANCY DISCOMFORTS

One of the nicest things you can do for your pregnant partner is to use your hands and fingers to make her pregnant body feel better. Massaging away her tiredness and fatigue can be a very sensual experience for you both. In addition, it can help relieve anxiety and help overcome depression. It can be very relaxing for her *and* for you! Acupressure, an ancient form of massage, can also help relieve common discomforts.

You can help out in a lot of ways. Sometimes a pregnant woman's aches are too far away for her to reach comfortably. At other times, her pains are completely out of reach. Sometimes your partner would just like to relax and let you do the work. Whatever her reasons for seeking your assistance, offer to do what you can to help her feel better, even if you don't have much of an idea about what you're doing. Your willingness to help her feel better may be as beneficial as the job you do.

One way to get started is to find some books or rent some videos that show various massage techniques. Some are available that focus mainly on pregnant

IN THE DOGHOUSE

Ignoring or minimizing your partner's fears can hurt both of you. A woman experiences lots of anxiety during pregnancy, from worrying about a glass of wine she had before she knew she was pregnant to being concerned her bag of waters will break in public. Although you probably won't be able to relieve all her worries, don't dismiss them out of hand. Listen to what the mom-to-be has to say, then try to reassure her that what she is feeling is perfectly normal.

women. You don't have to be an expert; take your time and concentrate on doing the best you can. As you practice the kneading and stroking techniques, you'll get better at doing them. Always use gentle pressure, and increase it only if your partner requests it. Immediately stop what you're doing if the mom-to-be says it hurts or doesn't feel good.

Before you begin, get some massage oil (you can buy this at a drugstore, specialty store or discount store) or a heavy moisturizer. Massage oil is often better to use because it stands up better to the friction of massage. Do a massage in a warm, quiet area, away from drafts. Don't massage immediately after a meal; wait at least an hour. Pillows and a blanket can help make your partner more comfortable and support her enlarging abdomen. Make sure your nails are short and free of rough edges, and your hands are clean.

Also keep in mind that a pregnant woman should not lie flat on her back after 16 weeks of pregnancy. Be sure your partner partially reclines or lies on her side while you massage her. Avoid putting any pressure directly on her abdomen.

When you practice acupressure techniques, do *not* use any oil. These techniques should also be done with the pregnant woman lying on her side. Pressure is applied with the thumbs or finger pads. You can also use your knuckles, the heel of the hand or a firm, blunt object, such as a pencil eraser. When you first begin, use light pressure; gradually increase it but keep the pressure at the level she requests.

My Mother-in-Law Said

If a wedding ring or locket dangled over a mother-to-be's belly spins in a circle, the baby is a girl. If it swings back and forth, it's a boy.

There's really only one test that will determine if your baby is a boy or girl—amniocentesis! Even though ultrasound can often predict a baby's sex, it is not foolproof. You might want to wait till after the birth to buy all those pink, frilly things for your little girl or to decorate your little boy's room with a sports theme, unless you have amniocentesis.

You Need Some TLC, Too!

If you're like many men, the demands of your job, helping to take care of the house, doing errands and caring for your pregnant partner may cause you some stress. There's nothing like a good back rub or a head massage to help *you* relax and enjoy your life more.

Tell your partner when you feel the need for some TLC—tender loving care. Ask her to rub your back or to massage your feet. What's good for her is also good for you. She can try some of the techniques described below, or together you can devise some relaxation techniques to relieve your tension.

A positive aspect for the pregnant woman in helping you relieve your tension and stress is that the activity is good for her hands, especially if they are swollen. Using her hands to rub or to massage you can help reduce her swelling—it's good for both of you!

A Back Rub Is Basic

Many women experience back pain during pregnancy. It's one of the most common discomforts women say they have. These pains are caused by relaxing ligaments that put added strain on the back muscles. A pregnant woman's overstretched abdominal muscles also put stress on the back as they attempt to support her upper and middle body.

Giving your partner a good back rub can work wonders for her. There are two techniques you can use to help relieve discomfort. Both are described below.

FOR A LOWER-BACK ACHE. Have your partner sit on a bench or stool, facing away from you. She should lean forward slightly. Stand at her back, to one side. Run one hand up her back, along the muscles of her spine. In one long, gliding movement done with your entire hand flat on her body, move your hand from her hip to the top of her shoulder. Repeat on each side several times.

Next, kneel behind your partner. Place both thumbs on the small bone at the base of her spine. With your thumbs, make small circles, alternating pressure from one thumb to the other. Let her be the guide to how much pressure you should apply.

If you want to try some acupressure, first apply heat or an ice pack to the upper-outer area of the buttocks adjacent to the spine. (You can find this point by having your partner find the indented area in the middle of her back, just below her waist.) Next apply firm, steady pressure with your fingertips or knuckles. Move the skin in small circles. (This technique may also help relieve the pain of sciatica. See the discussion below.)

FOR AN UPPER-BACK ACHE.   With your partner sitting at a table, resting her head on a pillow on the table, stand behind her. Place one hand on her shoulder. Using your other hand, in one long, gliding movement done with your fingers together and your entire hand flat on her body, stroke the middle of her back, moving up and over her shoulders. Make small circles along her shoulder blades with your thumb. Alternate shoulders, repeating several times.

Next, have her lift her head, still facing away from you. Reach around her, place one hand on her forehead and have her rest her head in your hand. With your other hand, rub up and down the back of her neck several times. Switch hands, and use your other hand to rub the opposite side of her neck.

When Her Legs Are Swollen
In addition to relieving discomfort, massage can help with swelling. If your partner has swollen legs, have her lie on her side on the sofa or bed. Place a pillow or two under her head. Sit by her feet, and place her legs in your lap. Begin on the leg that is on top. In one long, gliding movement done with your entire hand flat on her body, move your hand along her thigh, from her knee to her hip, on the front of her leg several times. Do the same movement on the back of her thigh. Be sure the pressure you exert is toward her heart, which helps move fluid out of her extremities.

Next, while gently pressing and kneading in a circular motion just above her ankle, begin making small circles up her leg toward her heart.

Lastly, put your hand under her heel, and lift her top leg a few inches off the sofa or bed. Move your other hand toward you from the tendon that extends from the back of her calf to her heel (the Achilles tendon). Alternate hands so you massage both sides of her leg.

When you have finished massaging one leg, have your partner roll over onto her other side so you can massage her other leg.

Sciatica Can Be a Real Pain!

Sciatica can be extremely painful, and massage can help. (See page 60 for information on sciatica.) Have your partner lie on her side on the sofa or bed, with her affected leg on top. Kneel next to your partner on the floor. Apply gentle pressure to the length of her leg in one long, gliding movement done with your entire hand flat on her body. Do this to the front of her leg, then the back of her leg. Start with the thigh, move to her lower leg and end with her foot. Include her buttocks in the massage.

BROWNIE POINTS

When your partner has trouble bending over because her large tummy gets in the way, offer to do some of the activities that she can no longer do comfortably. A few that come to mind—offer to tie her shoes, paint or clip her toenails, or ask her if she'd like you to shave her legs! (You need to be *very* careful when you do this last task.)

Next, lightly knead the leg with one hand while placing the other hand on the mom-to-be's hip to stabilize the leg. Repeat several times.

Lastly, place your thumbs on the back of her leg, at the top of the leg. Move the thumbs together down her leg. Next, in one long, gliding movement done with your entire hand flat on her body, move your hand along the entire length of the back of her leg. Finally, gently tap the back of her thigh, near her buttocks, with the back of your hand for 15 seconds.

Other Stress-Relieving Techniques

Some women love having their feet or hands massaged to help relieve swelling and to get their joints moving more easily. A foot massage can do more than just make your partner's feet feel good. When you massage her feet, you may help relieve headaches, boost her energy levels and aid digestion!

YOGA. Some yoga-type exercises can be fun to do together, and they'll help improve the mom-to-be's balance and flexibility. They can also help tone muscles. You may also benefit from doing them.

In the first exercise, stand about a foot apart, facing each other. Grasp each other's wrists. Breathing deeply, each of you should gently lean back as far as it is comfortable to do so. Hold this position for at least 10 seconds, then slowly come back to an upright position. Repeat several times.

In the next exercise, stand side to side, with your feet about 10 to 12 inches apart, your arms around each other's waists and your

---

Naming Your Baby

One way to begin bonding with your baby is for you and your partner to starting thinking about names for him or her. When you do this together, you strengthen the bond between you as a couple, and you begin to create a bond with your developing baby. A name gives the expected baby an identity and helps you feel closer to him or her.

Choosing a name for a child that he or she will have for the rest of his or her life can be a daunting experience, especially because you haven't met yet. However, there are some things to keep in mind when you are considering names for baby.

• Think about names that you like. You probably don't want to choose a name you don't like because you'll have to hear it forever!

• Try saying the name out loud. Is this a name that will sound good for a child *and* an adult?

• Choose a name with a definition that is meaningful to you or your partner.

• Consider a family name—by giving it to your child, you will honor other family members. If you don't want to use the same name, can you vary it?

• Be careful about choosing a unique or different name. Sometimes it's difficult to spell. Or it may be hard to pronounce. Will people (often children) make fun of the name?

• Think about words a name might rhyme with—are there some very negative words that could be rhymed with it that would embarrass your child?

(continued on next page)

(continued from previous page)

• The first name should complement the last name. Some believe the number of syllables in the first name should not be the same number as the surname. However, others like the sound of the same number of syllables for the first and last names.

• How might the name be shortened? Do you like it? For example, Edward may be shortened to Ed or Eddie.

• Pay attention to the middle name you give your child. What do the initials spell?

• Say the names you have chosen—first, middle and last—out loud several times to hear how they sound. Speak just the first and last names together. Yell it loudly, so you can hear how it might sound when you need to call to your child from a distance. (Trust us, you'll be yelling someday.)

• If you choose to give your child two middle names, think about filling out forms. In the U.S., this could be a problem because it's not usually done (in Europe and Great Britain this is an acceptable practice).

• Be aware of any family or religious customs that might prevent you from using a name.

hips touching. Have your partner lift her outside foot and place the bottom of it against the inner thigh of her other leg. Encourage her to breathe deeply while you support her in this position. Repeat several times.

In the third exercise, sit on the floor facing one another. Stretch legs apart, and touch the soles of your feet to the soles of your partner's feet. Holding each other's arms, breathe deeply for up to 60 seconds while you maintain the stretch.

HEADACHE RELIEF. Acupressure may help relieve headaches. Place your fingertips of your index finger and your middle finger on each of your partner's temples. Apply gentle pressure while you slowly move your fingers in small circles. Keep this up for about 60 seconds.

BONDING WITH YOUR BABY

Bonding with your baby is an incredible experience. *Bonding* is the process of becoming attached emotionally and physically to your baby. Most of the time it occurs after a baby is born; however, there are things you can do to bond with your baby now, during pregnancy.

It's usually easier for a woman to bond with her baby because she is linked to the fetus as it grows in her womb. It can be harder for a man to bond with his baby before birth, but you can do it. If you begin bonding with baby before birth, it'll be easier to continue after he or she is born. Ways to bond with your unborn baby include the following.

✓ Be involved in your partner's pregnancy.

✓ Try to be close physically and emotionally to the mom-to-be during pregnancy; this connection between you establishes a connection between you and your baby.

✓ Connect with your baby while it is still in the uterus. Make contact through your partner's tummy—talk to your baby, caress mom's tummy and "play" with baby.

✓ Place your hands on your partner's tummy when baby is moving so you can feel it.

✓ Go to prenatal visits with your partner.

✓ Take childbirth-education classes together.

We also cover ways to bond with your baby after birth. See pages 242–244.

6

You're Part of This Pregnancy, Too!

If someone told you a few months ago that when a woman gets pregnant the man is pregnant too, you probably would have laughed. However, now that you are a pregnant couple, you may be more understanding of how this can occur.

Supporting the mom-to-be by accompanying her to various prenatal tests and going to office visits may not seem like a lot to do, but it is. A woman wants to share the excitement of the developing fetus with her partner. She wants the help of her partner when she has difficulty getting around, and she needs his support when she has problems. Your support is *very* valuable.

Chapter Focus

To participate in making decisions about this pregnancy, you need to know about various tests your partner might have and why they're done. This chapter covers prenatal tests that are commonly performed and tests that are used in special situations. Each test is described so you will have an idea of what will occur, what test results may mean and how you can support your partner. At the end of this section, we provide you with information about some tests that may be done on the fetus during pregnancy and when labor begins.

It's also helpful to know why attending prenatal visits is important. We discuss what might happen at prenatal visits and what areas you and your partner might want to discuss with the physician at a visit.

AN IN-DEPTH LOOK AT PRENATAL TESTS

Tests are an important part of a woman's prenatal care; every test provides the doctor with information to plan the best course of treatment for a woman and her developing baby. Tests your partner takes can help reassure you both that your baby is doing well as it develops and that anything that might need to be done, can be done.

Early Prenatal Tests

When your partner goes to her first or second prenatal visit, the doctor will probably order a lot of tests. The tests that may be ordered, and why they are done, include:

✓ a complete blood count (CBC)—to check iron stores and to check for infections

✓ urinalysis and urine culture—to test for any infections and to determine the levels of sugar and protein in the urine

✓ a test for syphilis—to see if the woman has syphilis; treatment will be started if a woman is infected (this test is required by law)

✓ cervical cultures—to test for sexually transmitted diseases (STDs); when a Pap smear is done, a sample may also be taken to check for chlamydia, gonorrhea or other STDs

✓ rubella titers—to check for immunity against rubella

✓ blood type—to determine the woman's blood type (A, B, AB or O)

✓ Rh-factor—to determine if the woman is Rh-negative

✓ a test for hepatitis-B antibodies—to see if the woman has ever been exposed to hepatitis-B

✓ Pap smear—an early screening test for cervical cancer

✓ HIV/AIDS test—to determine if a woman has HIV or AIDS; it is not done routinely (the test cannot be done without the woman's knowledge *and* permission)

✓ AFP (alpha-fetoprotein), triple-screen or quad-screen tests— test done on a woman's blood to check for neural-tube defects, such as spina bifida, in fetus

Test results help the doctor determine what treatment may be necessary during this pregnancy or what actions might be necessary before another pregnancy is attempted. For example, if testing shows a woman has never had rubella (German measles) or she never received the rubella vaccine, she knows she needs to avoid exposure during this pregnancy and to receive the vaccine before her next pregnancy.

If your partner has difficulty having her blood drawn or she gets lightheaded or faint after blood is taken, you might want to accompany her to these tests. She may want your moral support, or she may appreciate it if you drive her to the tests, then take her home.

PELVIC EXAMS.   A pelvic examination is usually done at the first or second prenatal visit and again in late pregnancy. It is done early in pregnancy to evaluate the size of the uterus, to perform a Pap smear and to help the doctor determine how far along in the pregnancy a woman is. It is done again late in pregnancy because it tells the doctor many things, such as if the cervix is dilating and thinning.

Routine Tests Done at Every Visit

When you go to prenatal visits with your partner, you will note she is weighed, her blood pressure is checked and she provides a urine sample every time. These three simple tests provide a great deal of information. Gaining too much weight or not gaining enough weight can indicate problems. High blood pressure can be very significant during pregnancy, especially nearer the due date. By taking her blood pressure throughout the pregnancy, the doctor establishes what is normal for the mom-to-be. Changes in blood-pressure readings alert the doctor to potential problems. A urine sample checks for protein and bacteria in the urine, which can indicate problems.

As your baby grows, your partner is checked to see how much her uterus has grown since her last visit. The doctor also listens to the fetal heartbeat with a special listening machine, called a *doppler* or *doptone*. It magnifies the sound of the baby's heartbeat so it can be heard easily. It is possible to hear the baby's heartbeat

IN THE DOGHOUSE

Don't take offense if your partner asks you not to come to an office visit. She may be scheduled for a pelvic exam, or she may want to discuss something with the doctor that is private to her.

around the 12-week visit. You might want to find out when this will be done so you can be sure to attend that prenatal visit.

Why Do I Need to Know about the Tests My Partner May Have?

We provide you with detailed, comprehensive information about tests in this chapter to help you become informed about situations that might arise during pregnancy. It isn't necessary to know about every one of them; however, it's a good idea to have the information available, in case you need to find some answers. We believe that having the information at hand allows you to discuss a scenario with your partner, and it will help you formulate questions that you both may want to ask the doctor at a prenatal visit.

Ultrasound

An ultrasound exam may be one of the most exciting, fun tests you will have as a couple during pregnancy! Make every effort to be there. You'll enjoy being able to see your growing baby inside the mother's womb. Seeing baby moving may help make pregnancy and the baby more real for you.

Many doctors routinely perform ultrasound exams on pregnant patients, but not every doctor does them with every patient. The test enables the doctor to check for many details of fetal growth and development. (*Ultrasound, sonogram* and *sonography* refer to the same test.) Some doctors perform ultrasounds *only* when there is a problem.

In some cases, a doctor or technician will perform the test in the office at a visit, if the office has ultrasound equipment. If not, you and your partner may be sent to a lab where the test is performed. When the test is completed, results are usually discussed immediately with the couple if there is a problem. If everything appears normal, you and your partner will discuss results at the next prenatal visit.

An ultrasound can be done just about any time during pregnancy. The test is usually done at certain times in pregnancy to

---

Listen to Baby's Heartbeat at Home!

If you find listening to your growing baby's heartbeat fascinating, and you think you'd like to experience it more often than just at prenatal visits, now you can listen at home! You can rent or purchase a high-quality doppler to use in the privacy of your own home. These portable machines are small, lightweight and easy to use. Ask the doctor about where you can find one in your area. If you can't readily find a machine to rent or to buy, check the *Resources* section, page 261, for an Internet reference.

determine specific information. For example, when the doctor wants to check baby's size or to date the pregnancy, an ultrasound is most accurate in the middle of pregnancy.

Ultrasound gives a 2-dimensional picture of the developing baby by applying an alternating current to a device called a *transducer*. (In some areas, 3-dimensional ultrasound is being tested.) The transducer emits sound waves, then picks up echoes of those sound waves as they bounce off the baby; a computer translates them into a picture. This can be compared to radar used by airplanes or ships to create a picture of the terrain under a night sky or on the ocean floor.

Before the test, your partner may be asked to consume 32 ounces (1 quart; almost 1 liter) of water; this amount of water makes it easier for the technician to see the uterus. The bladder lies in front of the uterus; a full bladder pushes the uterus up and out of the pelvis area so it is seen more easily by the ultrasound. Be sure to ask about this; it is not necessary with every ultrasound.

REASONS FOR DOING AN ULTRASOUND. An ultrasound can help the doctor determine many things, including determining or confirming a due date, finding out how many fetuses there are and if major physical characteristics of

---

MEMORABLE MOMENTS FROM DR. DAD

Patty and Matt came to the office for an ultrasound at 20 weeks. Matt looked bored. Up to this time, he had not been too excited about the pregnancy, but he agreed to go to the ultrasound because Patty asked him to. They brought a blank videotape to record the ultrasound and gave it to the technician. The test is routinely done in a darkened room, and when the lights were turned on after the test was over, Patty could see how moved Matt was. There were tears on his cheeks, and he had to clear his throat. From that moment on, he was much more excited about, and involved in, the pregnancy. He showed the videotape of their baby's ultrasound to anyone who came to the house, including the washer repairman!

the fetus are normal. An ultrasound may be ordered to learn vital information about a fetus's brain, spine, face, major organs or limbs. The test can show where the placenta is, so it is used with other tests, such as amniocentesis. It can also provide information on fetal growth, the condition of the umbilical cord and the amount of amniotic fluid in the uterus.

If an ultrasound is done after 18 weeks, it *may* be possible to determine the sex of your baby, but don't count on it. It isn't always possible to tell the sex if the baby has its legs crossed or is in a breech presentation. Even if the technician or your doctor makes a prediction as to the sex of your baby, keep in mind that ultrasound prediction of fetal sex can be wrong.

OTHER FACTS ABOUT ULTRASOUND.   You and your partner may be able to get a videotape of your ultrasound; ask about it when the test is scheduled to find out if you need to bring a new, unused videotape. Most ultrasounds produce black-and-white photos you may keep.

The cost of an ultrasound varies. An average cost is about $150, but it can range from $100 to $300. With many insurance plans, ultrasound is an "extra" and not covered under the normal fee for prenatal care. Some insurance plans require preapproval for the test. Ask about cost and coverage *before* your ultrasound.

Amniocentesis

With amniocentesis, amniotic fluid is removed from the amniotic sac to test for some genetic defects and for other testing purposes. The test is usually done in a hospital setting, by a physician skilled in doing the procedure. You will probably want to accompany your partner to the test to offer moral support and to drive her home when she is finished.

Amniocentesis can identify about 40 fetal abnormalities. It can be used to screen for chromosomal defects, such as Down syndrome, and some specific gene defects, including cystic fibrosis and sickle cell disease. Amniocentesis may be performed to see if the baby of an Rh-negative woman is having problems. Toward the end of a pregnancy, it may be done to determine fetal lung maturity. Amniocentesis can also determine baby's sex. However, the test is not used for this purpose, except in cases in which baby's sex could predict a problem, such as hemophilia.

Amniocentesis is usually performed for prenatal evaluation around 16 weeks of pregnancy. Some doctors now do the test at around 11 or 12 weeks; however, this early use is considered experimental.

HOW THE TEST IS PERFORMED.   Ultrasound locates a pocket of fluid where the fetus and placenta are not in the way. Skin over the mother's abdomen is cleaned and numbed with a local anesthetic. A needle is passed through the abdomen into the uterus, and fluid is withdrawn with a syringe. About 1 ounce of amniotic fluid is needed to perform tests.

RISKS WITH AMNIOCENTESIS.   Although risks are relatively small, there is some risk associated with the procedure, including trauma to the fetus, placenta or umbilical cord, infection, miscarriage or premature labor. Fetal loss from complications is estimated to be between 0.3 and 3%. Discuss risks with the doctor before you and your partner decide whether she will have the test.

Some Specific Blood Tests that May Be Done

The tests discussed below are done by drawing blood from a pregnant woman, then testing the blood. They are performed because they provide you, your partner and the doctor with additional information; knowing the test is being done for this purpose may cause you and your partner some stress. You may want to accompany her to the test, if only to provide moral support.

ALPHA-FETOPROTEIN TEST.   The alpha-fetoprotein (AFP) test is a blood test done on the mother-to-be to help the doctor predict problems in the baby, such as spina bifida or Down syndrome. Alpha-fetoprotein is produced in the baby's liver, and it passes into a mother-to-be's bloodstream in small quantities, where it can be measured. The test is usually performed between 16 and 20 weeks of pregnancy. Test results must be correlated with the mother's age and weight, and the gestational age of the fetus. If AFP detects a possible problem, more definitive testing is usually ordered.

AFP can detect neural-tube defects, severe kidney or liver disease, esophageal or intestinal blockage, urinary obstruction, fragility of the baby's bones, called *osteogenesis imperfecta,* and Down syndrome. (AFP detects only about 25% of the cases of Down syndrome; if Down syndrome is indicated by AFP, additional diagnostic tests are usually ordered.) At this time, AFP is not performed on all pregnant women but is required in some states. If the test is not offered to your partner, discuss it with the doctor at one of her first prenatal visits.

One problem with AFP is a very high number of false-positive results. This means the results say there is a problem when there isn't one. Currently, if 1,000 women take an AFP test, 40 test results come back "abnormal." Of those 40, only 1 or 2 women actually have a problem.

If your partner has an AFP and the test result is abnormal, don't panic. She will probably have another AFP test, and an ultrasound might also be performed. Results from these additional tests should give a clearer answer. Be sure you understand what "false-positive" and "false-negative" test results mean. Ask the doctor to explain what each result can mean.

TRIPLE-SCREEN AND QUAD-SCREEN TESTS.   Tests that go beyond alpha-fetoprotein testing are available now to help a doctor determine if a fetus might have Down syndrome and to rule out other problems in the pregnancy. They are often referred to as *multiple-marker screening tests.*

The *triple-screen test* helps identify problems during pregnancy using three blood components: alpha-fetoprotein, human chorionic gonadotropin (HCG) and unconjugated estriol, a form of estrogen produced by the placenta. Abnormal levels of these three blood chemicals can indicate Down syndrome or neural-tube defects.

The *quad-screen test* is like the triple-screen but adds a fourth measurement—the blood level of inhibin-A, a chemical produced by the ovaries and placenta. This fourth measurement raises the sensitivity of the standard triple-screen test in determining if a fetus has Down syndrome. It can also predict neural-tube defects, such as spina bifida.

Chorionic Villus Sampling

Chorionic villus sampling (CVS) is used to detect genetic abnormalities; sampling is done early in pregnancy. The test analyzes chorionic villus cells, which eventually become the placenta.

The advantage of CVS is that the doctor can diagnose a problem fairly early in pregnancy. The test can be done at 9 to 11 weeks instead of 16 to 18 weeks, as with amniocentesis. Some couples choose CVS so they can make an early decision about the pregnancy. The procedure may carry fewer risks when performed earlier in pregnancy.

How the test is performed.   An instrument is placed through the cervix or through the abdomen to remove a small piece of tissue from the placenta. The procedure carries a small risk of miscarriage; it should be performed only by someone who has experience doing the test.

Because the test is usually done in a hospital setting, by a physician skilled in doing the procedure, you will probably want to accompany your partner to the test to offer moral support and to drive her home when she is finished.

Other Tests to Help Predict Problems

Various other tests are used to help predict problems in a baby before birth. We provide you with information so you know something about them if they are discussed at a prenatal visit or your partner wants to discuss them with you.

Glucose-tolerance test.   This test is done to check for gestational diabetes, which occurs only during pregnancy. The mother-to-be drinks a special sugar solution; then an hour later, blood is drawn to measure the level of sugar in the blood. In some cases, blood is drawn at additional intervals.

Group-B streptococcus (GBS).   Samples are taken from the expectant woman's vagina, perineum and rectum to check for GBS. A urine test may also be done. If the test is positive, treatment will be started or appropriate precautions will be taken during labor. This test is usually done near the end of the pregnancy.

GENETICS TESTS.   Various screening and diagnostic tests may be done to determine whether a growing fetus has certain birth defects. One of the newer tests is for cystic fibrosis. If you and your partner undergo genetic counseling, tests may be ordered for both of you. In other situations, the doctor will order tests if he or she determines they are necessary.

IMAGING TESTS.   There is no known safe amount of radiation from X-ray tests for a developing fetus. Your partner should avoid exposure to X-rays during pregnancy, unless it is an emergency. The medical need for the X-ray must always be weighed against its risk to the pregnancy. This warning also applies to dental X-rays.

Risk to the fetus appears to be the greatest between 8 and 15 weeks of pregnancy. Some physicians believe the only safe amount of radiation exposure for a fetus is no exposure.

Computerized tomographic scans, also called *CT scans* or *CAT scans,* are specialized X-rays that also involve computer analysis. Many researchers believe the radiation received from a CT scan is far lower than that from a regular X-ray. However, it is probably wise to avoid even this amount of exposure, if possible.

Magnetic resonance imaging, also called *MRI,* is widely used today. No harmful effects have been reported from its use in pregnancy, but pregnant women are advised to avoid MRI during the first trimester of pregnancy.

HOME UTERINE MONITORING.   Some women are monitored at home during pregnancy with home uterine monitoring. Contractions of a pregnant woman's uterus are recorded, then transmitted by telephone to the doctor. The procedure is used to identify women at risk of premature labor. Costs vary but run between $80 and $100 a day.

SPECIALIZED TESTS.   With *nuchal translucency screening,* a detailed ultrasound that allows the doctor to measure the space behind baby's neck is combined with a blood test. When combined, the results of these two tests can predict a woman's risk of having a baby with Down syndrome. An advantage of the test is that it can be done at 10 to 14 weeks, so the couple may make earlier decisions regarding the pregnancy, if they choose to do so.

Other tests that may be done include those described below. *Familial Mediterranean fever* is found in people of Armenian, Arabic, Turkish and Sephardic Jewish background. Prenatal testing helps identify carriers of the recessive gene so diagnosis can be made quickly in a newborn to avoid a potentially fatal medical problem.

Canavan's disease is most commonly found in people of Ashkenazi Jewish background. Canavan's disease screening can be combined with Tay-Sachs screening to determine if a fetus is affected.

Congenital deafness caused by the connexin-26 gene may occur if a couple has a family history of inherited deafness; this test may identify the problem before birth. With early identification, measures can be taken to manage the problem immediately after baby is born.

Some Less Common Tests

FETOSCOPY.   Fetoscopy enables a doctor to look through a fetoscope to detect subtle abnormalities and problems in a fetus. Because of advances in fiber optics, we are now able to look at a fetus or placenta as early as 10 weeks into its development. (Ultrasound cannot provide the same degree of detail.) This test is specialized and is usually recommended only if a woman has already given birth to a child with a birth defect that cannot be detected by any other test. If your doctor suggests fetoscopy, the three of you should discuss it at a prenatal visit. The risk of miscarriage is 3 to 4%. The procedure should be done *only* by someone experienced at performing it.

The test is performed by making a small incision in the mother's abdomen; a scope similar to the one used in laparoscopy is placed through the abdomen. The doctor uses the fetoscope to examine the fetus and placenta.

Because the test is usually done in a hospital setting, by a physician skilled in doing the procedure, you will probably want to accompany your partner to the test to offer moral support and to drive her home when she is finished.

PERCUTANEOUS UMBILICAL BLOOD SAMPLING (CORDOCENTESIS). Percutaneous umbilical blood sampling (PUBS) is a test done on the fetus while it is still in the womb. This test has improved the diagnosis and treatment of Rh-incompatibility, blood disorders and infections. The advantage of the test is that results are available within a few days; the disadvantage is it carries a slightly higher risk of miscarriage than amniocentesis.

Guided by ultrasound, the physician inserts a fine needle through a woman's abdomen into a tiny vein in the umbilical cord of the fetus. A small sample of the baby's blood is removed for analysis.

If there is a problem, a blood transfusion can be done, if it is necessary. This can help prevent life-threatening anemia that can develop if the mother is isoimmunized and the fetus has Rh-positive blood.

This test is usually done in a hospital setting, by a physician skilled in doing the procedure. You will probably want to accompany your partner to the test to offer moral support and to drive her home when she is finished.

FETAL FIBRONECTIN (fFN) TEST.   Fetal fibronectin (fFN) is a protein found in the amniotic sac and fetal membranes during the first 22 weeks of pregnancy. If a doctor believes a woman is going into premature labor, he or she may decide to test the woman's cervical-vaginal secretions. If fFN is present after 22 weeks, it indicates increased risk for preterm delivery. If it is absent, the risk is low and the woman probably won't deliver in the next 2 weeks.

The test is done the same way as a Pap smear is performed. A swab of cervical-vaginal secretions is taken from the top of the vagina, behind the cervix. Results are available from the lab within 24 hours.

TESTS ON BABY TO DETERMINE FETAL WELFARE

Various tests may be done to determine the well-being of your baby. Many of these tests are done on the mother-to-be but provide a glimpse of life inside the womb. You may want to accompany your partner to these tests.

Kick Count

Toward the end of pregnancy, your partner may be asked to record how often she feels the baby move. This test is done at home and is called a *kick count*. It provides reassurance about fetal well-being; this information is similar to that learned by a nonstress test. See the discussion below.

Your doctor may use one of two common methods. The first is to count how many times the baby moves in an hour. The other is to note how long it takes for baby to move 10 times. Usually the mom-to-be can choose when she wants to do the test. After eating a meal is a good time because baby is often more active then. This test is usually done at home.

Nonstress Test

A nonstress test is a simple, noninvasive procedure done around 32 weeks gestation or later; it is performed in the doctor's office or in the labor-and-delivery department at the hospital. This test measures how the fetal heart responds to the fetus's own movements and evaluates fetal well-being in late pregnancy. It is commonly used in overdue and high-risk pregnancies.

While she is lying down, a monitor is attached to your partner's abdomen. Every time she feels the baby move, she pushes a button to make a mark on the monitor paper. At the same time, the fetal monitor records the baby's heartbeat on the same paper.

If the baby doesn't move or if the heart rate does not react to movement, the test is called *nonreactive*. This doesn't necessarily mean there is a problem—the baby may be sleeping. In more than 75% of nonreactive tests, the baby is healthy. However, a nonreactive test might be a sign the baby is not receiving enough oxygen or is experiencing some other problem. In this case, the test will probably be repeated in 24 hours or additional tests will be ordered, including a contraction-stress test or a biophysical profile (see below).

Contraction-Stress Test

If the nonstress test is nonreactive (see the discussion above), a contraction-stress test (CST), also called a *stress test,* may be ordered to measure the response of the fetal heart to mild uterine contractions that mimic labor.

If your partner has had a problem pregnancy in the past or experienced medical problems during this pregnancy, your doctor may order this test in the last few weeks of pregnancy. If the mom-to-be has diabetes and takes insulin, your baby may be at some increased risk of problems. In that situation, the test may be done every week, beginning around 32 weeks.

In some cases, the doctor may order the nonstress test alone or order both the nonstress test and the contraction-stress test at the same time. (The contraction-stress test is considered more accurate than the nonstress test.)

This test is usually done in the hospital because it can take an hour or more and occasionally triggers labor. A nurse places a monitor on the abdomen to record the fetal heart rate. Nipple stimulation or oxytocin given intravenously in small amounts may be used to make the woman's uterus contract. Results indicate how well a baby will tolerate contractions and labor.

A slowed heart rate after a contraction may be a sign of fetal distress. The baby may not be receiving enough oxygen or may be experiencing some other difficulty. The doctor may recommend delivery of the baby. In other cases, the test may be repeated the next day or a biophysical profile ordered (see below). If the test shows no sign of a slowed fetal heart rate, the test result is reassuring.

> ### My Mother-in-Law Said
>
> *If the fetal heart rate is over 140, it's a girl. If it's under 140, it's a boy.*
>
> Different babies have different heart rates; a boy can have a high heart rate, and a girl may have a low heart rate. Don't depend on this method to determine baby's sex.

Biophysical Profile

A biophysical profile is a comprehensive test that helps determine the fetus's health status. The test is commonly performed in high-risk situations, overdue pregnancies or pregnancies in which the baby doesn't move very much. It's useful in evaluating an infant with intrauterine-growth restriction.

A biophysical profile measures five areas, which are identified and scored: fetal breathing movements, gross body movements, fetal tone, reactive fetal heart rate and amount of amniotic fluid. Ultrasound, external monitors and direct observation are used to take the various measurements.

Each area is given a score between 0 and 2. A score of 1 in any test is a middle score; a total is obtained by adding the five scores together. The higher the score, the better the baby's condition.

A baby with a low score may need to be delivered immediately. Your doctor will evaluate the scores, your partner's health and her pregnancy history before any decisions are made. If the score is reassuring, the test may be repeated at intervals. Sometimes the test will be repeated the following day.

Fetal Monitoring during Labor

In many hospitals, a baby's heartbeat is monitored throughout labor with external fetal monitoring or internal fetal monitoring. Fetal monitoring enables the doctor to detect problems early.

External fetal monitoring can be done before your partner's membranes rupture. A belt with a recorder is strapped to her abdomen to pick up the baby's heartbeat. *Internal fetal monitoring* monitors the baby more precisely. An electrode is placed through the vagina, into the womb, and attached to the fetus's scalp to measure the fetal heart rate. This test is done *only* after membranes have ruptured.

Fetal Blood Sampling during Labor

Fetal blood sampling is another way to evaluate how well a baby tolerates the stress of labor. Before the test can be performed, a woman's membranes must be ruptured, and the cervix must be dilated at least 2cm (about an inch). An instrument is passed into the vagina, through the dilated cervix to the top of the baby's head, where it makes a small nick in the baby's scalp. The baby's blood is collected in a small tube, and its pH (acidity) is checked.

Knowing the baby's pH level helps the doctor determine if the baby is having trouble or is under stress. The test helps the physician decide whether labor can continue or if a Cesarean delivery is needed.

Evaluating Fetal Lung Maturity

The respiratory system is the last fetal system to mature. Premature infants commonly experience respiratory difficulties because their lungs are not fully developed. Knowing how mature the baby's lungs are helps the doctor make a decision about early delivery, if that must be considered.

If the baby needs to be delivered early, tests can determine whether the baby will be able to breathe without assistance. Two tests used most often to evaluate a baby's lungs before birth are the *L-S ratio* and the *phosphatidyl glycerol (PG)* tests. Fluid for these two tests is obtained by amniocentesis.

Test to Determine Oxygen Levels

We can now monitor baby's oxygen *inside* the womb, before birth. Light measures the oxygen level in fetal blood, providing accurate answers as to whether baby's oxygen levels are in the safe range. This noninvasive approach, called *OxiFirst* fetal oxygen monitoring, is used during labor. A probe is placed inside the womb on baby's skin to measure the baby's oxygen level.

OFFICE VISITS CAN BE EDUCATIONAL AND INFORMATIVE FOR YOU BOTH

You may be wondering whether you really need to go to all the doctor's appointments your partner is scheduled to have in the coming months. We suggest you go with her whenever you can—attend as many visits as possible. You may not be able to go to every visit, but it's definitely worth it when you can. It can be very helpful to your partner, and it can be enjoyable for you.

Going to prenatal visits can make you feel more involved in the pregnancy and can bring you closer together as a family. You may have to rearrange your schedule or be creative with your time, but you'll probably benefit from going to as many office visits as you can.

Every woman feels differently about her partner's involvement in her pregnancy, so ask your partner how often she would like you to go to visits with her. You may be surprised that she may only want you there for something important, such as hearing the baby's heartbeat or for an ultrasound. There are many important reasons to go to visits, which are discussed below.

Be Sure to Ask Questions

The doctor and his or her staff are there to answer your questions and to provide you with help and reassurance during your pregnancy. If you or your partner forget to ask about something at an office visit, or a situation arises that you want to clarify, call the office. Ask to speak to the nurse if you want information, if instructions from the doctor are unclear or for any other reason. If she can't help you immediately, she'll find an answer.

The office staff and the doctor *expect* you to call. As a matter of fact, they would rather have you call about something and find out the correct answer than to have you ignore a situation that could become serious or to have you worry about something that is minor. So call when either you or your partner need information or assistance.

BROWNIE POINTS

Make up a list of questions you want to ask the doctor at a prenatal visit. Let your partner look over them, and discuss any that are important *before* you meet with the doctor. A discussion with the physician allows you to get specific answers to areas that are of concern to you, and it demonstrates to your partner that you are taking an active interest in the pregnancy.

Emotional Support

Going to prenatal visits together as a couple provides emotional support to you both and helps you experience the pregnancy together. It can help you share the highs and survive the lows of this miracle that is helping you become a family.

Physical Help

At various points during pregnancy, your partner's growing body size or the discomforts of her pregnancy can physically make it more challenging for her to drive a car, go up and down stairs or just get out of the house. Work together as a couple to help her get over these "rough spots."

You May Have Questions, Too

Pregnancy has ups and downs. You'll experience fun, exciting moments and sweat through anxious or nerve-wracking times. You may have questions about particular aspects of the pregnancy that

---

When to Call the Doctor

Don't rely on friends or family members for medical advice. When you need it, call the office. If your partner experiences any of the following signs or symptoms, call the doctor immediately. General warning signs include:

- vaginal bleeding
- severe swelling of the face or fingers
- severe abdominal pain
- loss of fluid from the vagina (usually a gushing of fluid but sometimes a trickle or a continual wetness)
- a big change in the movement of the baby or a lack of fetal movement
- high fever—more than 101.6F (38.7C)
- chills
- severe vomiting or an inability to keep food or liquids down
- blurred vision
- painful urination
- a headache that won't go away or a severe headache
- an injury or accident that hurts your partner or gives either of you concern about the well-being of your pregnancy, such as a fall or an automobile accident

are important to you. Attending office visits can help you find answers to your questions.

Decisions Must Be Made

As a couple, it will be easier to make decisions about labor, delivery, choosing a pediatrician and other situations if you attend visits together. It can help keep communication between you open, and it can help eliminate "When you see the doctor, ask her about . . ." or "Why didn't you ask him about . . . ?"

What If I Can't Make It to Every Visit?

We realize it may not be possible for you to go to every visit, so we've included some information on various visits that might be good to attend. This may help you decide which visits you don't want to miss.

✓ Go to a visit at various times throughout the pregnancy. Attend at least one office appointment in the 1st trimester of pregnancy.

✓ At the first visit (often around 8 weeks), the doctor often gives an overview of what lies ahead. A family history may also be taken at this time; it's helpful to be there to provide details of your family's health history.

✓ Another good early visit is at 12 weeks, when the fetal heartbeat can usually be heard for the first time. You may want to make that one!

✓ A visit during the second trimester clues you in to what may be happening at that time. Your doctor will also be able to give you advice on ways to help the mom-to-be during this time.

✓ At 20 weeks, many doctors perform an ultrasound. This test can be very exciting for both of you.

IN THE DOGHOUSE

Don't take the attitude that all the medical decisions about labor and delivery are your partner's to make. Listen to what your doctor says at prenatal visits, and ask questions about things you don't understand. Be willing to offer your opinion when it's asked for.

✓ Attend office visits if there are any problems or complications that need to be addressed.

✓ Toward the end of the pregnancy (especially the last 6 weeks), attend as many visits as possible. Use visits to discuss childbirth-education classes and plans for labor and delivery.

✓ Take your partner to visits when she needs physical help getting there, such as in bad weather or when she's not feeling well.

✓ Go with her when she has to have tests or procedures that are more serious than routine ones. She may need your moral support, or she may need you to take her home and care for her afterward.

BROWNIE POINTS

Be willing to take time off from work or other activities or to rearrange your schedule to go to prenatal tests with your partner if she needs your moral support or your physical presence.

Your Patience Is Appreciated

The people in the doctor's office know your time (and your partner's time, too) is important. They will try to get you in to see the doctor as soon as possible. However, plan for plenty of time at office visits, and be patient. Doctors who deliver babies have trouble controlling their schedules because they can't schedule when a baby will be born, except with some Cesarean deliveries. When you have your baby, you'll want the doctor to be with you!

If you ask for a late appointment or the last one of the day, expect to wait quite a while. This is often the busiest time in an obstetrician's office. You'll definitely spend time in the waiting room!

7

The Financial Realities of Parenthood

Are you feeling overwhelmed at the thought of being a good provider for your family? It can be a formidable task to prepare financially for the birth of your baby and beyond, especially when faced with the fact that in today's dollars, the estimated cost of raising your little bundle of joy to age 18 could exceed $200,000!

"How are we going to pay for all this?" is a common concern many fathers-to-be express. You may become more aware of your financial situation at this time because you start thinking about the costs associated with having and raising a child. You must consider *all* the costs—from the cost of the pregnancy and delivery to the costs involved in buying all the things you will need for baby. And you can't ignore costs that will come in the future—from child care to college!

Talk with your partner; together begin to explore your financial situation today and to think about what may come tomorrow. By considering your future, you can plan for almost any situation that might arise. Providing your child financial security while he or she is growing up is a goal most parents want to reach.

Chapter Focus

In this chapter, we explore many of the financial aspects of having a baby. We help you analyze your financial situation today and offer suggestions on ways you can improve it. We explain the importance of making a will. We look into the types of insurance you may have—from life insurance to medical-health insurance. We examine child-care costs and provide information on the tax savings of having a child. And we point out ways to save money for your child's use—from birth through his or her college education. Finally, we cover some of the information you might not realize you need to know that will affect your lives now and in the future.

EVALUATE YOUR SPENDING

Do you pay much attention to where your money goes and how much you spend as a couple? Some people know where they spend every penny. Others haven't a clue as to what their expenses are every month. It's important to have a handle on your spending. Why? Because having a baby means more expenses, so you may need to economize. If you don't know where you spend your money, it's harder to curb expenses.

Keep a Record for a Month

It's a good idea to evaluate your spending. To help you understand where your money goes and to identify areas where you may be able to cut expenses, keep a record for 1 month of everything you spend as a couple. Begin by listing all your fixed monthly expenses, such as mortgage or rent, utilities, insurance payments, car payments and any other expenses you have. Add to this figure the payments you make and the amount of interest you pay on credit-card debt, if any. (This is discussed in greater depth later in this chapter.)

Next, buy a small notebook, and carry it with you; have your partner do the same. Write down every expenditure (cash, check and credit card) you make, then transfer your expenses and your partner's into a notebook that you keep at home for this purpose. It may seem like a lot of work, but once you get going, it's fairly easy.

If carrying a notebook around is not for you, keep every receipt—for cash, check and credit-card purchases—then use the receipts to create one record of expenses. You may find it easier than writing things down at the time of purchase.

At the end of the month, sit down together and examine how you've spent your money. Compare the amount you spent with the amount of money you have coming in as a couple. How much do you have left over? When you understand where your money goes, you'll be able to make intelligent decisions about what changes you might need to make in your budget.

You may be surprised by how much you spend on things you don't think much about. But seeing your expenses in black and white can help you realize what your spending habits are. Some people find they can save money by cutting down on some expenditures.

Do You Need to Cut Expenses or Increase Your Income?

After examining your budget for the month, you and your partner may decide you both want better control of how you spend your money. With the baby coming soon, as a couple you may want to plan your spending so you'll be able to buy the things you'll need.

Look at where your money is going. Can you cut down on major expenses, such as using one car instead of two? Are some of the things you buy luxuries, not necessities? It may be in these areas that you can economize, if you find it necessary. For example, sell a car if only one is necessary and you have two. This saves money on car payments, insurance, gas and maintenance. For minor expenses, you might consider purchasing an expensive cup of coffee only once in a while instead of 3 or 4 times a week. Or instead of eating your lunch at a restaurant every day, consider taking your lunch 4 days a week and eating out on Fridays with friends or colleagues.

If you find it difficult to cut expenses, you may have to increase your income. Can you earn more money by working overtime, consulting during your off-hours or doing freelance work? If either of you works part-time, can you move to full-time work? Explore every way to increase your paycheck, if you can't cut expenses any further.

Whatever you do, make decisions together. It may be difficult to curb your spending, but as parents, it's important to provide financial security for your child. It's part of being a responsible parent. If you begin now, you'll have a handle on your present costs and those you will incur for baby's necessities. Knowing you are providing for your family may help you handle this big change in your financial situation more easily.

Get Control of Debt

After examining your spending, if you find you have incurred a lot of debt, this may be one area you need to address. If you are paying back loans, try to pay them off now. If credit-card spending and credit-card balances are out of hand, it's time to take control. It may take some work on your part, but it's worth it in the long run. You *can* do it. Try the following steps.

BROWNIE POINTS

Include your partner in any financial decisions you make for your family. After all, many of them directly affect her.

1. Get your credit-card statements out. Write down how much

you owe on each card. Next, find each account's annual percentage rate (APR), and compare them. These rates are probably not the same. Some may be low; others may be quite high. If you do not pay off your credit cards in full every month, the interest you pay can have an impact on your spending plan.

2. Decide which credit-card companies charge the highest APR. Make every effort to pay off the one with the highest APR first. If this means you have to send in only the minimum payment on your other credit cards until this is accomplished, then do it. Then take care of the balance on the next highest card. Do this until all your balances are paid off.

3. Keep only one credit card to use, and use it only when *absolutely* necessary. If you want to control your spending, one way to do it is to pay cash for as many purchases as possible. Pulling out your wallet and paying cash makes you more aware of how much you spend than just handing the sales clerk a piece of plastic.

4. If you have any loans (other than a mortgage), try to take care of them as soon as possible. If you can take care of loans within 8 to 12 months, do it. Many loans today allow you to pay them off early, without penalty. If you do this, you'll save the interest you would have paid, and you'll have more cash in hand every month.

5. Be willing to say "No" to unnecessary purchases. Before you buy something, think about your purchase. Do you really need it? Is it something you can hold off on? If you can avoid making unnecessary purchases, you'll help yourselves become debt-free.

> **Check the *Resources* Section for Information on Managing Finances**
>
> If you and your partner have tried to take control of your spending and find it hard to do, there are many sources of help and information available. Check the *Resources* section, which begins on page 261, for a list of agencies that can help you reach this important goal.

Saving for Emergencies and Other Important Needs

If your budget is stretched to its limits right now, how will you cope with an emergency? When something serious happens to you financially—loss of a job, unexpected financial costs, a major illness—will you be able to handle it?

Now is the time to make sure your family will have an emergency fund if it is needed. Most experts suggest enough money to cover living expenses for the entire family for 3 to 4 months. That includes mortgage or rent, utilities, food, transportation, loan payments, credit-card payments, child-care expenses—anything that needs to be paid to maintain your level of living.

If you do decide to establish an emergency fund, it's a good idea to be sure it is readily available. Put your money in a money-market fund or a higher-interest savings account so you will have access to it.

You may be fairly debt-free, but you may not have as much money in an emergency savings account as you would like. This is where your monthly-expenses record keeping can come in handy. It can help you see where you might be able to make adjustments in your spending habits, and it may give you some direction on how to do this.

Make the effort *now* to build this fund before baby's arrival. It could be very helpful if your partner cannot return to work when she planned or if you incur additional expenses you have not planned for.

Protect Your Credit Future

Make the most of your time and money by maintaining your good credit. It takes some work on your part, but it can pay off later. The following steps will help.

- Review your credit report once a year. This allows you to check for mistakes or fraudulent activity.
- If you find any errors or fraudulent activity, contact your credit-card companies and the credit bureau to make corrections.
- Use your credit wisely. Pay your account on time. Don't exceed your credit limits.
- Don't make purchases that max out your credit cards.
- Keep a record of all credit-card numbers and the telephone number of each credit-card company, in case you lose a card. You will be able to contact them quickly and cancel the card to protect yourself.

Start a Medical-Emergency Fund Now

If after checking your medical/health insurance you find some pregnancy-related costs are not covered, such as charges for the baby or the nursery, it might be wise to start a special savings account now to cover any out-of-pocket expenses. You'll have the money available when you need it, and you won't have to go into debt to pay for necessary care.

Be Financially Responsible

Becoming parents means you will have many new responsibilities. Being financially responsible may be one of your most important responsibilities. As a couple, you and your partner may not have planned how you spend your money. But with baby's arrival, your lives change, and this is one area that may require great changes.

If you begin to make adjustments now, you will feel secure and happy knowing you are providing your baby what he or she needs in life. Financial security will help you feel confident that you are beginning your parenting experience by addressing the needs of your growing family.

IT'S TIME TO MAKE YOUR WILL

Are you like nearly 60% of all Americans—are you "will-less"? The percentage is even higher for adults under age 35—almost 90% of people in this age group have not written a will! It's understandable; most people feel uncomfortable thinking about their own death and planning for it. But now is the time to rethink your procrastination, if you don't have a will. You need to take care of it *before* your baby's birth. And your partner should also write her will if she doesn't have one. It's important for both parents to have a will for the sake of their child.

If you have already written a will, kudos to you. Now is the time to check it for any changes or additions you may want to make. You may want to make various changes, such as renaming or updating beneficiaries, with the expected new addition to your family.

Name a Guardian

The most important aspect of a new or amended will is to name a guardian for your child. If something happens to you, your partner will take care of baby. However, what happens if something happens to you *both*, and your baby is left without parents? Who will care for him or her? Naming someone to care for your baby may be one of the most important things you can address at this time. Without a will that names a guardian, the courts decide who will care for your child.

There are a few things you must think about as you begin this process. Consider the following as you and your partner discuss, then decide upon, the person you choose for this important responsibility.

✓ Whom would you trust the most to care for your child?

✓ What is the age of this person?

✓ How good is his or her health?

✓ Is this person stable, financially and emotionally?

✓ Does he or she have a family, with children close to the same age? (This could be positive or negative.)

✓ Will your child grow up knowing this person?

✓ Does this person have the same values as you?

✓ Can this person handle the money you would leave for the care of your child?

✓ Who else could you choose if this person says "No" or couldn't care for your child in the future? (It's good to name at least two people in your will.)

AGREEING ON A GUARDIAN. How important is it for you and your partner to agree on a guardian? It's probably a good move to agree on one person and for each of you to name that person in your own will. This can save a lot of hassles if you both die at the same time. If you each name someone different, the courts will decide who, of the two people named, will care for your child.

After you have decided who you want to be the guardian of your child, ask that person. Don't put someone in your will as guardian without first asking him or her. He or she may have reasons you don't know about for not being able to accept this important role. It's a good idea to choose at least two people who could be the guardian of your child. Ask your first choice, and if he or she accepts, put the name in your will. Choose an alternative guardian (again, be sure to ask the person you select about it first, and tell that person that he or she will be named as the alternative).

Once the person has agreed to accept the role of guardian (or to be the alternate), put it in your will. If you believe you would prefer to have someone else handle the financial end of things for your child, you can also name a separate *property guardian*. This person's main responsibility is to take care of any financial assets you leave your child.

My Mother-in-Law Said

If a woman has her hair done just before baby's arrival, baby will have "good hair."

A baby's hair is determined by the genes he or she inherits from the parents. Nothing your partner does to her hair has any influence on baby's hair!

Who Will Inherit What?

When you draw up your will, you don't need to determine what will happen to property you and your partner jointly own. It passes directly to the other upon one person's death. Any assets you were required to name a beneficiary for pass to the beneficiary at that time.

So besides naming a guardian, what's the importance of writing a will? You need one to cover anything that you own *in your name only*. If you have separate savings, property or anything else that is not jointly owned, you must determine who gets what. Your will states this.

Many people believe that if they die without a will, their spouse inherits everything. This is not true. If you die without a will, the court will determine who gets what, based on state guidelines. If you are married, your wife and any children will probably divide everything between them. It's a good idea to make provisions for your spouse or another adult to handle the money until your child is old enough to do it on his or her own. If you are not married, a will becomes even more necessary to ensure your partner and child are taken care of.

Where Do We Go for a Will?

Some people will tell you that you don't need an attorney to draw up your will if you don't have a lot of property or many assets. They believe the do-it-yourself will kits available in some stores or on various computer programs cover all the bases. Some are fairly thorough; however, if you're not an attorney, you may be saving money now, but it could cost your child or your family later.

You want to make sure you dot all the *i*'s and cross all the *t*'s and that you have jumped through all the legal hoops so your wishes will be followed. The only way you can guarantee that is to use an attorney to oversee writing your will.

The cost of hiring an attorney to draw up a will can run from a few hundred dollars to a thousand dollars or more. However, we believe it's worth it to give you the peace of mind that your wishes will be followed regarding who cares for your child and who inherits or handles your money and assets.

In addition, you may want to have an attorney handle your will if you have a complicated life situation. For example, if you have substantial assets, and you believe your family would not respect your wishes, you may want to make sure your arrangements cannot easily be broken. If you have a child who is ill or one who will need care for the rest of his or her life, it's important to cover details of care arrangements in your will. If you are unmarried, an attorney

> **Protect Your Documents**
>
> Once you've made your wills, be sure you keep the originals in a safe place. If an attorney prepares yours, he or she will keep an original at the office. You might consider keeping a copy in a fireproof safety box at home.
>
> If you use a do-it-yourself will kit, keep your original document in a safe-deposit box at the bank. Keep a copy in a fireproof safety box at home. If you choose a relative to be the executor of your estate, you might also consider giving him or her a copy to have at hand.

IN THE DOGHOUSE

Don't put off making a will because it makes you feel uncomfortable to think about your own demise. A will proves to those you leave behind that you have taken an active interest in their welfare.

may be helpful in covering all the necessary aspects so your partner and child will inherit your assets.

If you do use a do-it-yourself will kit, you may want to ask an attorney to check it over for you when you are finished, to be sure you have covered everything. It may cost a little extra, but it could be well worth it if it saves your partner and your child problems in the future.

IT'S TIME TO CHECK YOUR INSURANCE

Now that you've made your will, it's time to arrange where some of the money will come from. This is most often provided through a life-insurance policy. While you are examining your life insurance, also take a look at the other types of insurance you have. You need to examine your life insurance, health/medical insurance, disability insurance and homeowner's or renter's insurance. Look at the coverage you have now, and determine what type of coverage you will need after baby's arrival. It's time to make any necessary changes!

When insurance of any type is provided by your employer or your partner's, check with the human resources (HR) representative for specific information about the insurance and its benefits. Don't overlook this important resource.

Life Insurance

If something happens to you, you want to be assured your child will be provided for and financially taken care of until he or she is an adult. It's important to have enough life insurance to cover raising your child through college. The U.S. government estimates it costs about $200,000 to raise a child born today through the age of 18. Add to that what the projected costs of college may be in 18 years. This is the amount of coverage that you should have. (Increase this amount as you add more children to your family.) You need coverage on your life *and* your partner's life to ensure there will be enough money to care for your child.

Pull out any existing policies, and sit down with your partner when you have enough time to go through all the details together. How much life-insurance coverage do you have? Do you have any coverage through your employer? How much is it? Most experts recommend 8 to 12 times a person's annual income to maintain a decent level of living for their children to grow up and to get through college.

If your partner is employed, find out if she has life-insurance coverage through her employer and how much coverage she has. If she has little or none, you may want to get a policy

> ### Insurance Is Costly!
> Most people don't realize how much of their annual income they spend on various types of insurance. If you have life insurance, homeowner's or renter's insurance, health insurance, disability insurance and car insurance, you may be spending 15% or more of your gross income on insurance premiums!

for her to help cover expenses should she die. If your partner doesn't work, consider getting coverage for her, if she doesn't have it already. (You may have to wait until after the baby's birth to purchase this insurance for her.) Determine how much child-care expenses cost in your area for a year, and add the cost of any help you would need in your home. A sum 10 times that yearly amount would provide you with a cushion to help provide care for your child.

WHOLE-LIFE OR TERM INSURANCE? Is your policy a whole-life policy or a term policy? With a *whole-life policy,* also called *permanent* or *cash-value insurance,* part of the premium you pay goes into a fund where it accumulates tax-free interest. You can draw on this interest in the future, if necessary. This is the type of insurance a person has when you hear about someone "taking out a loan" on his or her insurance.

With a *term policy,* you choose how long the insurance will cover you, such as 20 or 30 years; hence the word "term." Term is often the least expensive. You pay an annual premium based on your age at the time of purchase and the amount of coverage you select. It's less expensive to buy term insurance because all of your premium goes toward insurance—you're not putting any of it into a tax-free fund. In addition, it's easy to change your coverage as your family grows and your needs change. It's also important to look at how often you must renew it.

FINDING THE RIGHT INSURANCE FOR YOU.   If you discover you need to increase your life-insurance coverage, the best advice we can give you is, "Shop around!" Various companies offer different rates for the same coverage. You can contact some agencies, or check on the Internet. We list several websites in the *Resources*, beginning on page 270 where you can compare the cost of policies from several sources.

Insurance You *Don't* Need to Buy

With your baby on the way, you may be considering many types of insurance to purchase. However, there are several types of insurance you *don't* need that could cost you more than they pay back to your survivors. Be wary of the following types of policies.

• **Credit-life coverage.** This policy covers payments on your mortgage, loans or other debts in case of your death. It is more expensive than life insurance, and the money can *only* be applied to debt. In addition, a policy usually covers only one partner. If you want this coverage for you both, you have to buy two policies.

• **Policies that cover a disease.** With these policies, you're covering only one aspect of your health, such as cancer. It's wiser to buy a comprehensive health-insurance policy that provides coverage for many illnesses, diseases and conditions.

• **Life insurance on your child.** Unless your child will be earning an income—pretty rare for a new baby!—his or her death would not impact on your financial situation. And you don't need to "lock in insurability" of your child. It would probably be wiser to save for college the money that you'd pay in premiums.

• **Accidental death coverage.** This provides more money to your survivors in case you die in an accident, usually a car accident or a plane crash. The risk of dying in an accident is very low. If you feel you *must* have this type of insurance, check your credit cards. Some provide coverage in particular situations, such as your death in a plane crash, if you purchase your airline ticket with that card.

Medical or Health Coverage

One of the most important things you can do before your baby's birth is to review your health insurance. If your partner is employed, she may have coverage through her employer. If you are married and you are both covered, you probably have the choice of using the policy that has better coverage.

If your partner doesn't have health-care coverage, she may find it difficult to get coverage at this time. Many companies have a waiting period of 1 year before they will cover costs associated with childbirth. It might be a good idea to check to see if there is any type of coverage that might be available through various community programs. Or check out children's health-insurance programs in your state. Some provide medical coverage for a pregnant woman and her baby (after birth). Some programs are free; others are low-cost. These may be available to you even if you are both working.

There are quite a few things concerning coverage that you and your partner should think about when you examine your health-care insurance. Is the plan a traditional indemnity plan, in which you pay a deductible and/or a portion of all costs? Is the program a managed-care program, such as an HMO? Each provides different coverage. You and your partner will need answers to some very important questions about pregnancy coverage under the insurance plan you choose to use. If both of you work, you may have coverage under two policies. Family coverage under one policy might be a good choice, or consider which policy has the better coverage for one parent and the baby.

To get an idea of what is covered under your policy, talk to the people in the personnel department or the HR specialist. If that person cannot provide you with the answers you seek, you might consider calling the insurance company directly and speaking with someone there who can answer your questions. Some questions you may want to ask include the following.

✓ What type of coverage is it?
✓ Are there maternity benefits? What are they?
✓ Do maternity benefits cover Cesarean deliveries?
✓ What types of anesthesia do maternity benefits cover?
✓ What kind of coverage is there for a high-risk pregnancy?
✓ Is there a deductible? If so, what is it? How often is it paid?

✓ How are claims submitted?

✓ Is there a cap on total coverage?

✓ What percentage of costs are covered?

✓ Does coverage restrict the kind of hospital accommodations we may choose, such as a birthing center or a birthing room?

✓ What procedures must be followed before entering the hospital?

✓ Does the policy cover a nurse-midwife?

✓ Does coverage include medications?

✓ What tests during pregnancy are covered under the policy?

✓ What tests during labor and delivery are covered under the policy?

✓ What types of anesthesia are covered during labor and delivery?

✓ How long can mother and baby stay in the hospital?

✓ Does payment go directly to the healthcare provider or to us?

✓ What conditions or services are not covered?

✓ What kind of coverage is there for the baby after he or she is born?

✓ Is the pediatrician we have chosen covered?

✓ Is there an additional cost to add the baby to the policy?

✓ How do I add the baby to the policy?

✓ How much time do I have to add the baby to the policy?

Check your insurance for coverage of tests, procedures, medications and any other maternity and birth expenses. For example, some insurance companies do not cover routine ultrasound, so it's important to know this before one is scheduled. Some companies don't cover the new baby—you may be responsible for all of his or her hospital costs. Or the doctor you have chosen or the hospital you'd like to go to may not be covered. If your insurance doesn't cover all medical costs, you may need to start preparing for this as soon as you can.

Do You Have Disability Insurance? Do You Need It?

If you or your partner has an accident that requires you to take time off your job, disability insurance is good coverage to have. This insurance pays you a predetermined amount of money while you are disabled. Most employers provide some disability insurance, but *each working parent* should have enough insurance to cover between 65 and 75% of his or her income.

Your employer or your partner's employer may provide disability insurance through your place of work. The drawback to disability insurance through your employment is that coverage stops when you leave the

> ### Adding Baby to Your Policy
>
> Check your insurance policy *before* your baby is born to see what the time limit is for adding him or her to your health insurance. In some cases, the baby must be added within 30 days following the birth or no coverage will be provided.

job, and benefits are often fairly low. In addition, there is a difference, taxwise, between employer-sponsored policies and a policy you purchase on your own. If the company pays the premium, you will pay taxes on any money you receive. If you pay the premium, income you receive is tax-free.

If you decide to purchase a policy on your own, look for one that is guaranteed renewable and that cannot be canceled until you are 65. The best policies define "being disabled" as not being able to work at the job *you usually hold*. Some less expensive policies pay you only if you cannot do *any* type of work. Avoid these policies.

Check out the waiting period—many policies provided by an employer have a 30- to 90-day waiting period. Your partner's sick leave may not cover an extended period of time. This is where an emergency fund can be crucial. In addition, premiums may be lower if you choose a longer waiting period before benefits begin.

A WORD TO THE WISE. Have your partner check with her employer to see if the company provides disability coverage to pregnant women. In some cases, coverage begins if a woman has serious health problems during pregnancy or when her baby is born. Or coverage may begin after the baby is born.

Your Homeowner's or Renter's Insurance
Homeowner's insurance is a good investment to protect you and your family against financial losses from various disasters. Your policy

probably includes a liability portion to protect you from lawsuits and other claims; this can be important in the future if someone has an accident in your home.

Examine the coverage provided by your insurance policy. If you decide to have in-home child care, be sure insurance covers *anyone* who works in your home, even an occasional babysitter or weekly cleaning help.

If you do not own your own home (and thus do not require homeowner's insurance), check into a renter's insurance policy. This insurance protects you against the same type of loss as a homeowner's policy in a rental situation. It's good coverage to have.

THE COST OF CHILD CARE

Whether you or your partner will continue working outside the home after the baby's birth is one decision that many parents wish they didn't have to make. However, out of financial necessity, one parent staying home full-time is not an option for many families.

**MEMORABLE MOMENTS
FROM DR. DAD**

When I walked into the examining room, I could tell I had interrupted an important conversation between Alex and Hailey. They had their insurance forms in hand, and they were talking about various expenses. The look on Alex's face said, "What's this all going to cost us?" They had begun to realize that having a baby costs a lot of money. We discussed this important aspect of their pregnancy, and at the end of our prenatal visit, I introduced them to Lorraine, the insurance clerk for the office. At their next visit, Alex related that Lorraine had answered many of their questions and directed them to ask other questions of their human resources specialist at work. Both Alex and Hailey felt relieved to have answers to many of their questions. Now they could relax and focus on the pregnancy.

And every parent wants to feel secure in the knowledge that the care his or her child receives while the parents are at work is the best available. Also see the discussion of child care in Chapter 9.

You usually must pay federal, state and local taxes for your care provider, including Social Security and Medicare taxes. There are certain exceptions for withholding and paying taxes if the quarterly amount you pay to a provider is under a certain amount. Contact the Internal Revenue Service and your state's Department of Economic Security for further information. If the person works in your home, you may also need to pay Workers' Compensation and unemployment insurance taxes. Be sure you have homeowner's or renter's insurance to cover them while they work in your home.

The Cost of Child Care

Paying for child care can be a big-budget item in your household expenses. For some families, it can cost 25% or more of their household budget. The cost of infant and toddler care (through age 3) is the highest—it can range from $100 to $300 (or more) a week, depending on the type of care you choose. And the cost doesn't drop dramatically as a child gets older either—the average cost for a 4-year-old can be over $100 a week. In-home care can be more costly or less costly, depending on any placement fees and additional fees you negotiate based on extra tasks you want the caregiver to perform.

Public funding is available for some limited-income families. Title EE is a program paid for with federal funds. Call your local Department of Social Services for further information.

There are some other programs to help deal with child-care costs; they include a federal tax-credit program, the dependent-care-assistance program and earned-income tax credit. These three programs are regulated by

IN THE DOGHOUSE

Don't "wait until baby comes" to address various financial concerns. With a new baby at home, your spare time will be greatly limited. Take action now, while you have time and energy to devote to your research and study.

the federal government; contact the Internal Revenue Service at 800-829-1040 for further information, or visit their website at www.irs.gov. Of all the children eligible to receive federal child-care assistance, only about 12% actually receive it because programs are not fully funded at this time.

In some situations, a child may have special-care needs. If your baby is born with a disability or a health problem that needs one-on-one attention, it may be harder to find good child care, and it may cost more for that care.

Start Living on Your Adjusted Income Now!

If one of you decides not to return to work after baby's birth, as a couple you need to explore how you will live on one paycheck. It may help to start *now* to live only on the salary of the person who will be working.

> **BROWNIE POINTS**
>
> Seek professional advice about financial issues you don't understand. It's not a sign of weakness; it's a sign of intelligence!

If you both will return to work, find out how much child care will cost; it can be very expensive for an infant. Find out what child-care costs are in your area, and begin setting aside money to cover it.

The best way we have found to deal with either situation is to begin living on your adjusted income *now,* before baby's birth. Put the extra money in a money-market account to get a higher interest rate. You'll have a nice savings account when baby arrives, and you'll have adjusted your lifestyle to the costs you will incur and the financial changes you will be making.

CHANGES IN YOUR TAX SITUATION

Having a baby can have an impact on your federal and state tax bills. Because babies cost a lot of money to have and to raise, it's important for parents to explore all the ways they can save when paying taxes. In this section, we discuss tax credits and other deductions you may be eligible for.

Review Your Withholding

One of the first things you can do is to review how much money is being withheld each pay period from your paycheck and from your partner's. You may want to wait until after baby is born to change your withholding, or you may want to think about adjusting your withholding now to reflect what that amount will be after your baby's birth. Be careful about changing your withholding if your baby is due close to the end of the year. If you adjust your withholding for the current year and baby doesn't make an appearance until after the new year, you may have some problems, taxwise. Talk to an accountant or a tax preparer if you have questions and concerns.

Don't spend any extra money. Put it in a savings account so you'll have it to use for various situations (maybe an unplanned-for emergency or extra costs incurred with baby?) that arise for your family. After baby arrives, keep saving the money.

Expanded Child Credit

Today, a family can reduce its tax bill by $600 for every child under age 17 in the family. (This reduction will rise to $1,000 by 2010.) This is in addition to the $3,000 personal exemption (in 2002) for each family member, which will increase every year. However, this credit begins to phase out when a family's adjusted gross income reaches a certain point and disappears for families who reach a higher financial level. Check with an accountant or tax preparer if you have questions.

To claim this deduction for your baby, your child *must* have a Social Security number, so be sure to get one early. (You'll need it for other reasons, too, as we discuss in following sections. See the discussion of how to get a Social Security number on page 162.)

Child and Dependent Care Tax Credit
(Child-Care Expenses)

Beginning in 2003, parents can claim a federal tax credit of up to 35% of eligible child-care expenses, depending on their combined income. If both parents are working, even if only part-time, child-care expenses of up to $2,400 a year for one child (a total of $4,800 for two or more) may be deducted if the child-care provider has a valid tax ID number (a Social Security number or a tax ID number). The number must be provided when you file your tax return. At this time, credit can be taken for care of children up to age 13 or for children older than 13 who are physically or mentally disabled.

Dependent-Care Reimbursement Accounts
Many companies now allow parents to set aside part of each pay-check for child-care costs. A benefit of this plan is that the money is

---

Is It Worth It to Return to Work?

You may wonder whether it's worth it financially for your partner (or you) to return to work after your baby's birth. You can do some calculations to help you come up with an answer. First, add up the following to find your total "working cost":

- cost of child care
- cost of formula (if mom cannot breastfeed) and duplicate equipment between home and child care
- tax liability of second income
- cost of travel to and from work
- cost of meals eaten out, dry cleaning, clothing and other necessary things
- cost of any "treats," such as eating out, buying convenience foods, having someone clean the house

To determine the cost of not working:

- Add together your take-home pay and benefits.
- Deduct total working costs.
- Divide this number by the total number of hours you spend away from home. This gives you a figure that represents how much you are making for each hour you are away from home and baby.
- Be sure to account for extras, such as the cost of insurance now provided by the employer.
- The bottom-line figure could surprise you.

not taxed. However, be aware that if you take advantage of this program, you *cannot* take a Child and Dependent Care tax credit, as described above.

If your company offers this program, talk with the human resources specialist about it. Find out how much money you would save with this plan, and compare it to how much money you could deduct from your taxes with the Child and Dependent Care tax credit. If you are still uncertain about the benefits of either plan, discuss it with an accountant or tax preparer.

Flexible Spending Accounts

You might also consider establishing a flexible spending account (FSA). An FSA is a method by which you or your partner, as an employee, can set aside part of your income in a separate account, maintained by your employer, to pay for qualifying medical expenses, including co-pays, insurance and other medical expenses. The decision of the amount to set aside is made *before* the year begins; any money unused at the end of the year is forfeited.

An FSA is a pretax benefit. For example, if you make $30,000 per year and designate $2,000 for an FSA at the beginning of the year, you will be taxed only on $28,000.

Unfortunately, an FSA is employer-driven, which means the employer must offer it as a benefit. As an individual, you cannot start this account on your own.

SAVING FOR YOUR CHILD'S FUTURE

It's always a good idea to set money aside to use solely for your child, so you have a fund to meet unexpected emergencies or to take care of various costs as the child grows up. One goal may be to pay for a college education; that is discussed in the section that follows. In this section, we discuss ways to set aside some money for your child that may be used for other things.

There are several ways to invest money for your child. The more risk you are willing to take, the higher the possibility of return on your investment. But a higher return also means you have a higher

risk of losing your money. You may want to choose a safer investment. You and your partner should work together to decide what
works for you and your baby.

It's a good idea to start a savings account for baby's future. Add
to it regularly; make it a part of your family budget. As your child
grows older, you can encourage him or her to add money to the account. This helps teach the child the value of saving and may help
establish good saving habits. You don't have to save a lot of money
every time you make a deposit. The key is to start early and to be
consistent—save a little every month or every paycheck.

Gifts from Others

When your baby is born, you will probably receive lots of gifts and
presents. Many will be useful with a new baby at home. Or people
may have no idea what you need and may ask you for suggestions.
When family members or friends ask what they can get for baby,
you can always mention baby's "savings fund." It's not rude,
gauche or out of line to suggest they donate money to your child's
account.

Baby's Bank Account

Open a savings account at your local bank or credit union soon after baby arrives. Put any money into this account that baby receives
as gifts. Add to the account whenever you can. As baby grows older,
add gift money or earned money to the account. If you begin the
saving habit early, the money can grow into a nice amount for your
child's future use.

U.S. Savings Bonds

If people don't feel comfortable putting money into your child's account, suggest they buy a U.S. Savings Bond for the child. They are
readily available at most banks and as a payroll deduction. Bonds
can be purchased in amounts as low as $25, and interest is exempt
from state and local taxes (but not federal taxes).

Bonds are a very safe investment because they are guaranteed by
the federal government. The interest or yield they pay is usually

competitive with bank CDs (certificates of deposit), but no tax is paid on the interest until the bonds are cashed in.

There are various types of U.S. Savings Bonds available, such as "I" bonds; the *I* stands for inflation. They may pay a slightly higher rate than other government bonds. The bonds you may be more familiar with are the Series EE bonds, which often pay a lower interest rate. However, the yield of these bonds is adjusted every 6 months.

Buying U.S. Savings Bonds may be an ideal way for grandma to put a little money aside for baby. Or an aunt or uncle who wants to contribute to baby's savings may find purchasing these bonds as a birthday present every year an easy way to do it.

Mutual Funds

Mutual funds, also called *custodial accounts,* can be another good avenue for investing for your child's future. Many funds are set up so you can put a little away every time you save. Quite a few are tailored to get you started saving this way because they require low initial investments (about $500).

If the mutual fund is held in the child's name (with a parent also on the account), you may receive a tax break on the savings. In most cases, interest paid on these investments is taxed at the children's rate of 10%, not your tax rate. This can be a big savings for some families.

It's not too early to investigate these types of savings accounts. Your child will actually receive more money if you save early in life, even if it's only for a limited number of years. The later you start, the less opportunity the money has to earn interest, so less money overall is earned. Also see the discussion of *Custodial Accounts* below.

SAVING FOR COLLEGE

It's a fact you'll soon realize—your baby will grow quickly. As unbelievable as it may seem now, it won't be long before he or she is old enough to go to college. In addition to the life-changing (for everyone) event of your offspring leaving home, you may be faced with the life-challenging experience of paying for it all!

A college education can drain the savings of parents who have not planned for it. With the cost of some 4-year educations at a private college exceeding $125,000 *today*, imagine what this cost will be when your child is ready to head off to school in 18 years! Some predictions are that it may cost as much as a *quarter of a million dollars* to attend a private college or university by the time your child is ready to start college.

What can you do about it? The best solution we can offer is to start *right now* to save for your child's education. There are quite a few ways you can do this; we explore them below.

The 529 Accounts

The 529 savings program was named for the section of the 1996 tax law that created it. Under this law, there are two ways you can save money for your child's college education. The first is the *college-savings plan*, which allows you to save money to be used at any college or university in the country. The second plan is the *prepaid college-tuition plan*, which allows you to pay for in-state tuition at a public university in your state.

These plans may offer state residents additional tax benefits. However, not all states offer additional benefits. Check with an accountant or tax preparer if you have any questions.

Most 529 plans are not run by individual states but by professional managers chosen by the state. With the college-savings plan, you can usually pick the investment option that interests you most. You can choose an investment plan, in almost any state, even if your child may not go to school there.

If you have more than one child, you must set up a savings plan for *each* child. Money saved in a 529 plan does *not* pass to the child at a given age; savings remain under control of the person who opened the account.

If you choose either of these plans, it's wise to start saving early in your child's life, especially with the prepaid-tuition plan. With college costs rising nearly every year, the sooner you start putting money into one of these plans, the greater return you'll receive on your money.

Below are discussions of both plans. Also see the box on page 160 for information on redeeming money saved under a 529 plan.

THE 529 COLLEGE-SAVINGS PLAN. This 529 plan is often referred to by its more common name, *college-savings plan.* It is a state-sponsored savings plan that allows you to save up to $305,000 to use for tuition and other educational expenses.

The plan provides tax-free growth of the money invested, professional management and high-contribution limits. Anyone can contribute to the plan, regardless of their relationship to the child.

With this plan, you choose one of the investment options provided by your state or the 30 states that allow nonresidents to invest. The money you save can be used at an accredited college or university *anywhere* in the United States.

The interest rates and the maximum amount that can be invested vary from state to state. The money grows tax-deferred and can be tax-free if it is used for school expenses. When taxes are paid on the money, they are paid at the child's tax rate, which will probably be lower than yours. In addition, the money doesn't need to be used by a specific time, so it can be used by the child at a later date, such as for graduate school. If the child does not need it or chooses not to attend school, it can be used by another family member, such as a sibling or cousin. *You* can even use the money for educational purposes! However, money can *only* be used for education at an accredited institution—it cannot be used for other activities or expenses. One drawback to this type of savings is that you have little or no choice in how the money is invested.

THE 529 PREPAID-TUITION PLAN. A prepaid-tuition plan is a second type of 529 plan and is offered by 18 states at this time. This plan helps parents pay for tuition at in-state public universities. However, some plans also allow you to transfer some or all of those assets to a school outside your state.

With a prepaid-tuition plan, in-state tuition to a state university is covered, in addition to fees, books and supplies. Sometimes room-and-board costs are also covered, if the student is enrolled at least half-time. You pay current tuition rates, to be used when your child goes to college. In essence, a current year's tuition rate will cover the cost of 1 year of school when your child enrolls in 18 years. If you decide to use this plan, begin investing early to take advantage of lower college costs.

Savings are guaranteed to increase in value at the same rate as the college costs. If your child decides to go to a different school, you can transfer some or all of the value of the plan to a private or out-of-state school. At this time, money is free from federal taxes when you withdraw it for school expenses. This tax-free status only applies to withdrawals made through 2010; however, most experts believe this tax break will be extended by Congress after 2010. Money can be used only for school expenses. Check with an accountant or tax preparer for additional information.

Can You Get Your Money Back from a 529 Plan?

The good news about this prepaid-tuition plan is that the money *can* be redeemed if the child doesn't need it for school. A parent or donor remains in control of the 529 money; if it is not needed because of scholarships or because the child does not go to college, the money can be "pulled back" by the parent or donor. (There is no penalty if the account is not used because the beneficiary dies, becomes disabled or receives a tax-free scholarship.) The person who redeems the money is taxed on the interest earned over the years, and a 10% penalty could be applied on the earnings, unless an exception is met. Check out the website www.savingforcollege.com for additional information.

Custodial Accounts

In the past, many parents have chosen custodial accounts as a way to save money for their child's college education. Children under 18 years old cannot usually own securities outright, so a plan of this type is set up to save money for a child. A custodial account may contain stocks, bonds and/or mutual funds.

A parent (or someone else) can invest in the child's name and still maintain control over the assets. The adult maintains control of the money until the child comes of age, usually 18 or 21, depending upon your state laws. At that time, the child becomes responsible for the account and any money in it, and can spend it any way he or she wants to, without having to consult anyone.

An advantage to this type of account is that a parent, relative or friend can each contribute up to $10,000 a year without having to pay a gift tax. Another advantage is that the money can be used for other things, besides education, that benefit the child.

Yearly earnings on this type of account are taxed differently from many other investments. Until a child is 14, he or she can earn $750 a year tax-free. The next $750 of earnings is taxed at the child's rate; any annual earnings above $1,500 are taxed at *your* tax rate until the child reaches the age of 14. When the child reaches 14, all of the earnings are taxed at his or her rate.

A disadvantage of a custodial account is the impact it can have on financial aid; it can actually *reduce* the amount of financial aid a child can receive. Most current formulas require a student to use from 25 to 35% of their own assets to pay for college costs each year before any financial aid will be granted. If a custodial account is large, the child will be required to use the money in the account before receiving financial aid.

Coverdell Education Savings Account (Education IRA)
Another type of savings account is the Coverdell Education Savings Account, which can be set up through a bank, credit union or online investment company. This plan used to be referred to as an *Education IRA*. The account allows you to make yearly nondeductible contributions in your child's name to a trust established for your child. Investment return may be higher than that paid on regular savings accounts because, similar to a custodial account, money may be invested in mutual funds and other holdings and can be invested for a longer period of time. Money can be used for *any* educational expenses, including primary school, secondary school and college expenses.

The contribution isn't tax-deductible, but the money accumulates tax-free, and it is not taxed when money is withdrawn from the account to pay for educational expenses. If the child doesn't use the IRA, it can be transferred to a sibling. Earnings should be spent before the child reaches age 30; however, any money that is not spent can be transferred to a minor sibling or a child of the person the trust was set up for.

Contributions to this type of account are limited to a total of $2,000 a year. Other family members or friends *cannot* open separate Coverdell accounts for the child. Because the amount you can deposit is limited, growth is also limited. In addition, you cannot contribute to a Coverdell account and a state plan (either type) in the same year.

SOME OTHER CONSIDERATIONS

As responsible parents, you and your partner want to take care of as many financial details as possible before baby's birth and soon after baby's arrival. Below are some other financial issues that you might not be aware of that you can address now or immediately after baby is born.

Baby's Social Security Number

It's important to request a Social Security number (SSN) for your child as soon after birth as possible. A Social Security number is needed for many things, such as opening a savings account for your child, buying stocks or bonds, or to claim your child on your taxes. While your partner is in the hospital, she may be given the necessary forms to fill out. She should take advantage of this service. However, understand that the hospital will *not* send the forms in for you—that is your responsibility! Be aware that turn-around time can be as long as 14 weeks.

If your partner is not given the form in the hospital, call the Social Security Administration and request one. Their toll-free number is 800-772-1213.

What Is Your Partner's Plan for Maternity Leave?

It's a good idea for your partner to discuss maternity leave with someone in authority where she works. She should sit down with her supervisor, the HR person and co-workers, if necessary, and discuss her plans and expectations about leaving work and returning to her job. She should be aware that some decisions may not be made until after baby's birth, such as when she will be back at work, because she cannot predict how everything will go for her. She may feel pretty fit and want to return earlier than expected. Or she may have a difficult delivery or a C-section and need to take more time off than she planned.

Different companies have different maternity-leave policies— policies can range from a short, unpaid time off to several months off, with full pay and benefits. Paid leave is usually covered by disability insurance. If your partner is considering saving as much of her vacation and sick days as she can to extend her maternity leave, she should discuss this plan with her employer.

Your partner should also check out what her maternity-leave rights may be, as granted under the Family and Medical Leave Act (see pages 82–83). She should be aware that, by law, she can't be questioned about her intentions regarding returning to work. But do encourage your partner to discuss her plans for taking time off fairly early, so plans can be made to cover her job.

Plan to Shop Smart

Because we are discussing the financial aspects of becoming parents in this chapter, we want to touch upon how you can begin to plan *now* to buy *later* what you will need for baby. We discuss preparing for baby in depth in Chapter 9 but address it here

> ## BROWNIE POINTS
> You and your partner are probably not the first ones at your place of employment to go through a pregnancy. You should each ask your employers about policies, resources, options and plans that are available to help you out. Talk with others at work to find out what experiences they have had in similar circumstances.

so you can think about how and where you will shop, what you want to buy and how much money you plan to spend.

It's a good idea to budget baby costs now, while you are still a little removed from the actual buying experience. Decide that you won't let these costs eat up your budget. While it's nice to have the best of everything for your baby, you don't always need it. Buy secondhand equipment, or borrow items from friends or family (as long as everything meets current safety standards). Shop many different types of stores, and don't forget to check out what's available on the Internet.

Rent a Safe-Deposit Box

It might be a good idea to look into renting a safe-deposit box, if you don't already have one. You can find them at banks and credit unions; the annual cost is fairly reasonable.

Use your box to store important documents for your family. These can include your marriage certificate, birth certificates, insurance policies, wills, Social Security cards, stock certificates, bonds,

---

Protect Your Social Security Numbers (and Baby's Too)

You may have been asked in the past, and you will probably be asked in the future, to supply your Social Security number (SSN) for various reasons, such as when you fill out forms, get a driver's license or for other reasons. We suggest you *not* give your SSN to anyone who doesn't need it. Your employer and your bank need it—there are few reasons for others to have it. Why the warning? Because when someone has your SSN, it's easier to steal your identity. We speak from experience. Safeguard your number, your spouse's number and your child's number.

When someone requests your SSN, ask them why they need it. If they can't give you a valid reason, other than "because . . .," give them your driver's license number. Is your driver's license number your Social Security number? You should be allowed to request another number instead of your SSN at your state motor vehicle department; use that number when filling out forms. It's for your own financial safety!

property deeds, valuables you don't need access to very often, such as jewelry, and any other items you want to protect. Make a list of everything you put in your safe-deposit box, and make copies of important documents to keep in a fireproof box at home. One or both of you may also consider keeping copies at your office.

When you rent the box, be sure *both* of you sign up for it, and that you are each provided a key. Be sure you can each have access on your own—that both of you don't have to go to the box together—in case there is a situation that allows only one of you to go to the box, such as an accident or death of either of you.

If One of You Decides to Stay at Home
Under recent revisions to the federal tax code, stay-at-home parents are gaining some new rights. At this time, higher limits for retirement savings have gone into effect. The parent who chooses to stay at home to raise a child can now save more in a retirement account in his or her own name. The amount you can now save is $3,000; that amount increases to $5,000 by 2008. Pretax 401(k) savings limits are also on the rise. Check with an accountant or tax preparer for further information.

8

If There Are Pregnancy Problems

Pregnancy and birth have been occurring for a *long* time, nearly always without complications or problems. Most pregnancies are usually problem-free, and the 9 months of waiting by a couple are a time filled with anticipation and happiness. The pregnancy progresses without medical problems, the mother-to-be's health is not greatly affected by how her body changes and adapts, and she gives birth to a healthy baby boy or girl. However, in a few cases, there *are* problems, and these problems commonly affect both partners.

You may not want to read this chapter unless you and your partner are faced with one of these challenges. If you are, you may be grateful to have this information available. Its purpose is to provide you with knowledge so you and your partner can discuss a problem, and how it might be handled, with the doctor.

The ways you help your partner cope with a problem during pregnancy can draw you closer together. You are a *very* important part of the pregnancy, and your support can be essential to having a healthy baby. If problems occur, you will realize just how important you are to your partner and your growing baby. This may be a part of the pregnancy when you can be of greatest help to your partner. Try to be positive and supportive if one of these conditions occurs in your pregnancy.

Some problems, such as gestational diabetes and pregnancy hypertension, are not unusual and occur in many pregnancies. They may cause no noticeable discomfort for the mom-to-be. But they are always important and must be monitored for the good health of your partner and baby.

If you or your partner have questions, don't be afraid to ask for help. Call the doctor or go to prenatal appointments to discuss your concerns. Although you or your partner may believe it's easier to get advice or information from family members or friends, *don't* rely on them for medical advice. Your doctor has probably dealt with similar situations many times. The answers he or she gives you will be right for your pregnancy. Another good resource for information is the doctor's nurse or assistant. Often he or she will have more time to talk with you and may be able to reach you sooner than the doctor.

Chapter Focus

In this chapter, we cover some of the more serious problems that can occur during a pregnancy. We don't go into a lot of detail about each problem; the doctor will discuss particulars with you if a problem occurs. Our goal in presenting this material is to give you ideas on ways you can support and help each other during this stressful time.

DO YOU NEED TO CALL THE DOCTOR?

You and your partner may be unsure what might constitute a serious problem during pregnancy, and you may not know when it is appropriate or important to call the doctor. If your partner experiences any of the following signs or symptoms, call the doctor immediately. General warning signs include:

✓ vaginal bleeding

✓ severe swelling of her face or fingers

✓ severe abdominal pain

✓ regular tightening or cramping (contractions) of the uterus

✓ loss of fluid from the vagina (usually a gushing of fluid but sometimes a trickle or a continual wetness)

✓ she feels a big change in the movement of the baby or a lack of fetal movement

✓ high fever—more than 101.6F (38.7C)

✓ chills

✓ severe vomiting or an inability to keep food or liquids down

✓ blurred vision

✓ painful urination

✓ a headache that won't go away or a severe headache

✓ an injury or accident that hurts her or gives either of you concern about the well-being of the baby, such as a fall or an automobile accident

Whenever either of you has a question that concerns the mom-to-be's health, call the doctor's office! They won't be annoyed—they answer these types of questions every day. You and your partner are the patients, and office staff would rather answer *every* question you have than to have an expectant mother who has a serious problem not call the office because she "doesn't want to be a bother."

There may be times when your partner will want you to make a telephone call to the doctor's office for her. That's OK. It is one way you can help and support her.

Once you make the call, don't be surprised or offended if the doc-

> ## IN THE DOGHOUSE
>
> Don't put off calling the doctor for advice or information if you believe your partner might be having a problem. Sometimes dealing with the problem *immediately* is necessary so a situation doesn't become more serious.

tor or nurse asks to speak directly to your partner, not to you. Communication is better, questions are more easily answered and information clearer when data does not have to be relayed from your partner to you to the doctor then back to your partner. You have been very helpful in making the call and getting someone on the line who can help. It's OK for you and your partner to both be on the telephone together, too.

WHEN THE NEWS IS NOT GOOD

When a pregnancy problem occurs, there is the chance that the outcome will not be what you expected, problems are greater than first believed or your hopes as a couple for a perfect baby are dashed. If you and your partner are faced with this situation, it may be harder to deal with than you might imagine. No one ever thinks that this situation will happen to them.

Our best advice to you, if this happens, is to make every attempt to deal with it *together*. Rely on one another for support during these stressful times. Allow yourselves time to grieve over your loss—whether it be the loss of your baby or the loss of your expectations for a perfect baby. A complication during pregnancy can be overwhelming for both of you. This is a time to take care of your partner and yourself.

You're Part of the Pregnancy

If problems do arise, keep in mind that you are part of the pregnancy, and you should be involved in making any important decisions. Don't leave decisions to your partner and the doctor; after all, it's your baby, too. Your willingness to talk about a problem and to help your partner examine all aspects of it demonstrate how important the pregnancy is to you. One of the greatest gifts you can give your new family is to take an active part in any decision-making process. When it's all behind you, you and your partner will be glad you did it together.

Include family members, if you choose to do so, and ask for their help, encouragement and support. If necessary, consider seeking outside support, such as a counselor or your minister, rabbi or priest, to help you through this ordeal. Friends and family members often want to help, but you may not welcome their attention at this time. Let them know if you need space.

You can help out by answering the telephone and screening calls. You may also want to limit visitors, if your partner asks you to do so or if you don't feel like dealing with people. Take care of your partner during this difficult time. You may want to ask a friend or family member to do the same for you.

You may need help with kids, if you have other children. This can allow you more time with your partner.

Many couples have said that some of their fondest memories from pregnancy come from adjustments they had to make in their lifestyles. Many of these changes became a part of their life together, even after their baby was born.

PREGNANCY PROBLEMS YOU MAY ENCOUNTER

In this section, we discuss some pregnancy problems that might occur. For the doctor to deal with a problem, he or she must know about it. That's why it's important for your partner to go to every scheduled prenatal visit. Her pregnancy progress can be followed, and any problems can be taken care of if they appear.

Bleeding during Pregnancy

Bleeding during pregnancy doesn't always mean there is a problem. Always advise the doctor about any bleeding; he or she may want your partner to have an ultrasound. An ultrasound won't stop the bleeding, but it may provide reassurance. About 20% of all women bleed sometime in early pregnancy. It is not uncommon for a small amount of bleeding, called *spotting,* to occur after your partner does any heavy physical activity or following intercourse.

Bleeding later in pregnancy raises concerns. If your partner experiences any bleeding at this time, call the doctor *immediately.* The problem may not be serious, but it must be evaluated.

SUPPORTING YOUR PARTNER.   Your partner may be advised to rest in bed, but there is no surgery or medicine that will stop bleeding. The doctor will make treatment decisions based on the pregnancy history. Attending a prenatal appointment to discuss the problem together can help. Your partner may ask you to call the doctor's office or go to the next prenatal appointment with her. If the bleeding

---

**MEMORABLE MOMENTS
FROM DR. DAD**

Elaine's ectopic pregnancy was physically and emotionally very difficult for her and Pete. They had been anticipating the birth of their baby, and loss of the pregnancy was unexpected. At the hospital, after the surgery, they both said they didn't know if they wanted to try for another pregnancy. I told them that it was normal to feel that way and to give themselves some time to grieve over their loss. I encouraged them to come to the office together in a few months, and we would talk about the future. At that visit, I reassured them that I believed they could try to get pregnant again, and I had every reason to believe that they would be successful. Two years later, it was an emotional and exciting experience to share in the birth of their twin daughters, Amy and Anne. Elaine and Pete were ecstatic that they were normal, healthy babies.

occurs following intercourse, she may want you present so you can discuss it together with the doctor.

Ectopic Pregnancy

An ectopic pregnancy, sometimes called a *tubal pregnancy,* is not common; it occurs only about once in every 100 pregnancies. It occurs when a fertilized egg implants outside the uterine cavity, most often in a Fallopian tube. One of the most common signs of ectopic pregnancy is pain; if pain is severe and causes you or your partner concern, call the doctor.

Diagnosing an ectopic pregnancy can be difficult and may require a few tests and some waiting. Tests include ultrasound, a quantitative HCG test and laparoscopy (a type of minor surgery). It may take days or even weeks to make a definitive diagnosis.

SUPPORTING YOUR PARTNER.   An ectopic pregnancy cannot be carried to full term. The pregnancy cannot be moved from the tube into the uterus. Surgery is almost always required to correct the problem. In some cases, it can be treated with a medication called *methotrexate.* This treatment is not available everywhere and cannot be used if the tube has ruptured.

In the case of an ectopic pregnancy, the pregnancy is lost. You both will probably be very sad and upset if this situation occurs. Work together to deal with your grief.

In addition, ectopic pregnancies often require surgery. If your partner has surgery, she will need your help and support while she recovers. She has lost the pregnancy, and she has had surgery. Your physical and emotional support during this stressful time will be critical to her.

If Your Partner Falls

A fall is the most frequent cause of minor injury during pregnancy. Fortunately, a fall usually doesn't cause serious injury to the fetus or mother. Movement of the baby after a fall is reassuring. A possible problem after a fall may be indicated by bleeding from the vagina, a gush of fluid from the vagina indicating rupture of membranes or severe abdominal pain.

If your partner falls, contact the doctor; the expectant mother may require attention or monitoring. If she has a very bad fall, the doctor may advise monitoring the baby's heartbeat or order an ultrasound of the mother-to-be for further evaluation.

SUPPORTING YOUR PARTNER.   A fall can be traumatic and frightening to a pregnant woman. She may be worried that she hurt the baby or that something is wrong with her. Your reassurance and support during this time is essential. You may have to check around your home to see if some preventive measures can be put in place. Offer to do jobs or chores that put her at risk of falling.

Gestational Diabetes

Some women develop a type of diabetes that appears *only* during pregnancy; it is called *gestational diabetes*. The condition is triggered when the usual hormone changes of pregnancy, combined with dietary factors, result in higher blood-sugar levels. High blood-sugar levels can result in a larger baby, making delivery more difficult, or baby may have a higher risk of birth defects, such as heart problems.

Gestational diabetes affects about 10% of all pregnancies. After pregnancy, nearly all women with gestational diabetes return to normal, and the problem disappears.

If the doctor finds an abnormal level of sugar in your partner's urine during routine tests (it's one reason the mother-to-be's urine is checked at every office visit), other tests will be done. Pregnancy diabetes is diagnosed with specific blood tests.

SUPPORTING YOUR PARTNER.   One of the best ways to treat gestational diabetes is with a good nutrition plan. Under the guidance of a dietician, a nutrition plan of three small meals and three small snacks is devised to limit the amount of food eaten at any one time. If your partner eats the wrong food, or too much food at one time, it can cause her blood sugar to rise.

You can still eat your meals together. Her meals will be smaller, and she may have to eat earlier or later than you usually do, but with a little planning, you can do it.

Help your partner by choosing foods that are healthy for her (and you!) to eat. Avoid sugars and sweets; keep fats to a minimum. Avoid artificial sweeteners. Each of her meals should contain milk, protein, fruit, vegetables, grains and a limited amount of fat. This nutrition plan is probably good for you, too. Snacks should contain a starch and a protein; the final snack of the day should also contain milk and a fat serving to help keep her sugar level constant during the night.

My Mother-in-Law Said

If a pregnant woman looks at something ugly, her baby will be ugly.

Every woman sees something ugly during pregnancy. If this were true, every baby would be ugly. (And there are *no* ugly babies!)

Hypertension during Pregnancy

Hypertension is another illness some pregnant women must deal with. (Hypertension is also called *high blood pressure.*) Most women who are hypertensive during pregnancy do not have high blood pressure when they aren't pregnant, and the problem usually disappears after the baby is born. Other women enter pregnancy with the problem.

When a woman experiences hypertension, the uterine blood vessels that supply the developing baby with nutrients and oxygen are constricted. This constriction can slow fetal development. Hypertension also increases the risk of placental abruption (separation of the placenta from the wall of the uterus before delivery).

Hypertension may lead to other problems; about 20% of all women who experience high blood pressure *before* pregnancy develop pre-eclampsia. About 25% of the women who develop pregnancy-induced hypertension develop pre-eclampsia.

The condition is treated with bed rest (see pages 183–185), increased fluid intake and avoiding salt and sodium-heavy foods. Medications to lower blood pressure may be prescribed if these changes don't work. Women who do not respond to these measures may have to be hospitalized.

SUPPORTING YOUR PARTNER. Help your partner avoid foods that contain a lot of salt and sodium. Support her in her efforts to drink a lot of fluid. Having her blood pressure checked on a regular basis is a good reason for your partner to keep all of her prenatal appointments.

If your partner is advised to rest in bed, be as helpful as you can. Ways you can do this are described in the section on bed rest later in this chapter. Help her follow the instructions given to her by the doctor. Make it possible for her to rest in bed by helping out and by not encouraging her to do things that are contrary to the medical advice she has been given.

Miscarriage

A *miscarriage* is the loss of a pregnancy before 20 weeks of gestation. (The loss of a pregnancy after 20 weeks is called a *stillbirth*.) The embryo or fetus is delivered before it can survive outside the womb.

Having a miscarriage is an emotional experience for any couple. Many couples mistakenly blame themselves when a miscarriage occurs. It isn't anyone's fault, so don't blame yourself or your partner.

We usually don't know why a miscarriage occurs; it can happen for many different reasons. The most common reason for early miscarriage is abnormal development of the embryo. Research indicates that more than half of all early miscarriages have chromosomal abnormalities. Outside factors, such as radiation and some chemicals (drugs or medications), may cause a miscarriage. In some cases, the union of a couple's sperm and egg results in genetic abnormalities that cause a miscarriage.

The first warning sign of a miscarriage is bleeding from the vagina, followed by cramping. Call the doctor immediately if your partner experiences this! Unfortunately, there is little your partner, you or the doctor can do to stop a miscarriage from happening; there is no surgical technique or medicine available that can stop a miscarriage.

SUPPORTING YOUR PARTNER. Most physicians recommend bed rest and decreased activity. Some prescribe the hormone progesterone, but not all doctors agree with its use. Ultrasound and blood tests may help the doctor determine whether a miscarriage will occur, but you may have to wait and see. In nearly all cases, the miscarriage will occur, regardless of anything you do.

This can be a very traumatic time for you both. Your partner will need your support, and you will need her support. Share your feelings about the loss and sadness you may be feeling. Don't blame each other for the problem. It is very common for one or both of you to feel responsible for a miscarriage.

This is an important time for you to support your partner and for her to support you. Reassure her that miscarriages frequently happen, and it's not her fault. It is hard for a couple to endure the loss of a pregnancy; feeling guilty about it is an unnecessary burden.

Problems with the Placenta

The placenta carries nourishment and oxygen from the mother-to-be to the developing baby, and it carries away the baby's waste products. Problems occasionally develop with the placenta, including *placenta previa, placental abruption* and *retained placenta*.

PLACENTA PREVIA.   With placenta previa, the placenta covers part or all of the woman's cervix. The placenta may separate from the uterus as the cervix begins to dilate (open) during labor, which causes heavy bleeding. Placenta previa affects about 1 in every 200 pregnant women during the last trimester of pregnancy. With placenta previa, the baby is more likely to be in a breech position. For this reason, and to avoid bleeding, a physician will almost always perform a Cesarean delivery. Signs and symptoms of placenta previa vary, but the most characteristic symptom is painless bleeding.

IN THE DOGHOUSE

If you experience a loss during this pregnancy, don't try to hold it inside you. You *need* to grieve to be able to move on. If you don't grieve, you may never fully recover from your loss.

SUPPORTING YOUR PARTNER.   If the doctor determines your partner has placenta previa, she will have to curtail certain activities. Most physicians recommend avoiding intercourse and not traveling, in addition to avoiding pelvic exams. Placenta previa can be a very serious problem and can result in heavy bleeding. If your partner is given instructions about her activities related to placenta previa, be supportive and help her follow the advice.

PLACENTAL ABRUPTION.   Placental abruption occurs when the placenta separates from the wall of the uterus before birth. Normally it does not separate until the baby's birth. Separation before birth can be dangerous for mother and baby.

Placental abruption occurs about once in every 80 deliveries. Its cause is unknown. The major symptom of placental abruption is heavy bleeding from the vagina. If bleeding is severe, the woman may go into shock because of blood loss. Other symptoms, such as pain or severe cramping, may also be present. In some cases, ultrasound may help diagnose the problem.

The most common treatment of placental abruption is delivery of the baby. However, the decision of when to deliver the baby varies, based on the problem's severity. Sometimes a Cesarean section is necessary, but each case is handled individually.

SUPPORTING YOUR PARTNER.   We know that maternal smoking and alcohol use may increase the risk of placental abruption. If your partner smokes cigarettes or drinks alcohol, encourage her to stop both activities (it's also advisable for many other reasons). Cocaine use may also cause placental abruption. Placental abruption can be frightening because there is the possibility of serious complications. This is a time when your support is critical. It is also important to follow instructions from medical personnel. Your partner may need to stay in the hospital or to curtail certain activities, such as going to work. She'll need your help, so be there!

RETAINED PLACENTA.   Sometimes there are problems delivering the placenta after the baby is born. Usually the placenta separates from the implantation site on the uterus a few minutes after delivery.

When the placenta or part of the placenta does not do this, we call it a *retained placenta*.

The most significant problem with a retained placenta is severe bleeding after delivery. If the placenta does not deliver on its own, the doctor may attempt to remove the placenta in a procedure called *dilatation and curettage (D&C)*. If the placenta is attached through the wall of the uterus, it may be necessary to remove the uterus by performing a hysterectomy; however, this is rare.

SUPPORTING YOUR PARTNER.   With a retained placenta, there is often a lot of bleeding; this can result in anemia. Anemia means a low blood count, which can result in fatigue and a lack of energy for your partner. It may be necessary for her to take iron supplements. In severe situations, a blood transfusion may be considered. Anemia from a retained placenta may result in a slower, more difficult recovery. Your partner may need more help from you for even the most routine tasks, like getting out of bed. This is an opportunity for you to pitch in and help out.

Pre-eclampsia

The condition of pre-eclampsia was once called *toxemia of pregnancy* or just *toxemia*. This problem can be a serious complication and occurs *only* during pregnancy. Pre-eclampsia may develop after the 20th week of pregnancy, though most cases occur after 30 weeks. Left untreated, it poses a serious threat to mother and baby.

Fortunately, most cases of pre-eclampsia are mild and treatable. With mild pre-eclampsia, blood pressure is slightly elevated. (Hypertension is discussed above.) The only other obvious symptom of mild pre-eclampsia might be swelling of the legs, hands and face.

Keeping all prenatal appointments is the best way a woman can reduce the risk of developing this condition. With the help and co-operation of the pregnant woman and her partner, the doctor can usually treat pre-eclampsia before it becomes serious.

Certain signs indicate a worsening condition. Call the doctor *immediately* if your partner has pre-eclampsia and develops pain under the ribs on the right side, has a headache, sees spots or notices other vision changes.

For a mild case of pre-eclampsia, the doctor will probably order bed rest until your partner's blood pressure stabilizes or she delivers the baby. She will be advised to drink lots of water and to avoid salt and foods containing large amounts of sodium. In some cases, the pregnant woman is given medication to lower her blood pressure.

If pre-eclampsia worsens, the mom-to-be may be admitted to the hospital for bed rest and observation. Blood tests may be done. The developing baby is also monitored and evaluated with tests, such as a biophysical profile, or a nonstress test may be done.

ECLAMPSIA.   Fortunately, pre-eclampsia does not usually get worse, but if it does, it can quickly progress to a serious condition called *eclampsia*. Eclampsia is accompanied by seizures or convulsions, and a woman can go into a coma. (A *seizure* is a loss of body control, such as passing out, and often includes twitching or shaking. A *convulsion* is a severe seizure.) Either a seizure or a convulsion could cause harm to the expectant mother or her baby.

Your partner may be given medication to protect against seizures, including magnesium sulfate, or antiseizure medicines, such as phenobarbital, may be prescribed. She may also be hospitalized for close monitoring.

> **BROWNIE POINTS**
>
> If problems arise, accompany your partner to prenatal visits to discuss the situation with the doctor. It will be easier if both of you have the same information; you won't have any miscommunication about what is happening.

If these measures don't help and your partner's condition doesn't improve, the baby may need to be delivered to protect the expectant mother from serious complications, including convulsions, stroke, liver damage and kidney damage. It's important for you to take an active part in the decision making.

SUPPORTING YOUR PARTNER.   As we advise with gestational diabetes, help your partner avoid foods that contain a lot of salt and sodium. Support her in her efforts to drink a lot of fluid. If your partner is advised to rest in bed, be as helpful and supportive as you can. Ways you can do this are described in the section on bed rest. If your partner's condition worsens, and she is admitted to the hospital, let her know you are willing to do whatever she needs to support her. Ask her what she would like you to take care of—there may be tasks she was planning to do before baby's birth that you may have to handle. If she is told she can't work, help her understand and accept the necessary changes.

Premature Labor and Preterm Birth

In some situations, a pregnant woman will show signs of premature labor, which can lead to preterm birth of the baby. *Preterm birth* refers to a baby born more than 4 weeks early; it is also called *premature birth*. About 10% of all babies are born between 34 and 36 weeks gestation; most are normal and healthy.

However, delivery much before this time may result in problems for the baby, especially if it is born before 32 weeks gestation. Preterm birth of a baby can be dangerous because the baby's lungs and other organ systems may not be fully developed and ready to function on their own. In most cases, it is better for both mother and baby if premature labor is halted. Premature delivery increases the risks of problems for the mother-to-be *and* the baby.

If your partner experiences premature labor, it is important for the doctor to try to stop the contractions. Most recommend bed rest and increased fluids as the first step. Medications may be prescribed later. Why is bed rest prescribed first? It often works to help end premature labor. Before we had medications, bed rest was the *only* treatment for premature labor. It is still often successful in halting premature labor.

There are some medications available that the doctor may use to try to stop premature labor, depending on your partner's pregnancy history. These medications relax the uterus and decrease contractions. Even if medication is prescribed for your partner, she will probably be advised to rest in bed. Medications that relax the uterus and decrease contractions include magnesium sulfate, beta-adrenergics and sedatives or narcotics.

SUPPORTING YOUR PARTNER.   If your partner is advised to rest in bed, be as helpful as you can. Ways you can do this are described in the following section. Sometimes it is helpful to realize that every day the baby stays inside the uterus is a day you won't have to visit the intensive-care nursery!

BED REST

Bed rest is ordered for a woman to improve her chances of giving birth to a healthy baby. A woman may be advised to rest in bed when certain conditions threaten the baby's or mother's health. The three most common reasons a woman is ordered to rest in bed are premature labor (which can lead to preterm birth), pre-eclampsia and placenta previa.

Today, one in five women spends at least 1 week in bed during pregnancy. If the condition is severe or she is unable to rest in bed at home, hospitalization may be advised.

Why bed rest? First, lying down takes the pressure of the baby's weight off her cervix, which can help when a woman experiences premature labor. Second, resting on her side maximizes the blood flow to her uterus, which brings more oxygen and nutrients to the baby. She may be allowed to alternate between sides, but she *cannot* lie on her back. Lying on her back puts too much pressure on the vena cava and decreases the blood supply to the baby.

Bed rest can seriously disrupt a couple's routine. Your partner may not be able to work, and she may have to curtail other activities; changing routines can be stressful. Staying in bed may be hard for your partner, but remind her it is better to rest at home than in the hospital!

Ask the doctor what your partner can and cannot do while she is on bed rest. Sometimes a woman isn't allowed to get out of bed except to eat, go to the bathroom and go to prenatal appointments. At other times, bed rest may be less restricted. A woman may be able to sit up or be a little more active for part of the day. She may also have to take medication.

Bed rest is often ordered near the end of pregnancy, and most women have so much to do before baby's arrival! It can be difficult for your partner to rest in bed. It may not be much fun for you, either, to have to assume more responsibilities as you get ready for baby's arrival. And it's *definitely* not very much fun if the doctor advises abstaining from sex as a part of bed rest.

Supporting Your Partner

Try to stay positive if your partner must rest in bed. This is good advice for both of you! The goal of resting in bed is a healthy baby and a healthy mom. If your partner feels upset or anxious over this development (it's a normal reaction), remind her that she's doing it to give your baby the best possible start in life.

There are some things you can do that might help your partner accept her confinement a little more easily. Keep her company when you're at home. It can get very lonely staying in bed all day long by yourself. Encourage her friends and family members to call or to stop by for a visit, if your partner feels up to it. If they offer to pitch in and help around the house, let them! Most people are happy to help out. Tasks they might do include grocery shopping, light cleaning, laundry, child care or making a meal.

Take over household chores. Fretting about a dirty bathroom or unwashed dishes can add to your partner's anxiety. At the same time, remind her that you can only do so much, so she will understand your home may not be as spotless as she would like.

If you're thinking about getting a gift, choose something that will help her deal with the long hours she must spend in bed. A new CD, rented videos,

BROWNIE POINTS

If either you or your partner are having any problems dealing with a situation, consider talking with someone who has knowledge and experience in the area. Sometimes talking with someone who is not directly involved helps a great deal. Your doctor's office can recommend someone who can help.

pretty stationery and stamps, a new book or books on tape can help her pass the time.

EMERGENCY SURGERY DURING PREGNANCY

Emergencies occur, even during pregnancy. When a woman is pregnant, a medical emergency must be dealt with in a way that is best for her *and* for her developing fetus. Sometimes surgical procedures are necessary. Some common reasons for surgery during pregnancy include gall-bladder removal, appendicitis, ovarian cysts, broken bones and dental emergencies.

Anesthesia or pain medication may be necessary for a surgical procedure. Ask the doctor to keep its use to a minimum. It is best for your partner and the baby to avoid general anesthesia in the first trimester and whenever else it is possible. If general anesthesia is required, doctors will monitor the baby closely throughout surgery.

In an emergency situation, the doctor will make every attempt to safeguard the health of mother and baby. If you are faced with this type of problem, make decisions together, along with the doctor. Understand that there are emergencies requiring surgery, such as appendicitis or broken bones, that need attention now and can't wait until the pregnancy is over.

9

Preparing for Baby's Arrival

You and your partner are probably getting pretty excited thinking about and preparing for your baby's arrival. Pretty soon all the waiting and anticipation will be over, and you'll begin your new life as a family.

In these weeks of preparation, you may have a lot of things you want to do, such as painting baby's room, buying nursery furniture, getting a *new* car seat (this is one of the *most* important and few pieces of new equipment we recommend you buy). It's fun to take care of these things together, although we suggest the mom-to-be avoid freshly painted walls and furniture.

You may have other concerns, too, such as taking childbirth-education classes and practicing what you learn at home. If you choose to be your partner's labor coach, this may take extra preparation. These issues are covered in Chapter 10. Issues you *don't* want to avoid addressing at this time include selecting a pediatrician and choosing child care. You and your partner should both be thinking about these two matters. Why now? To be prepared!

It's best if you can choose your baby's doctor *before* baby's birth so the physician can examine baby at the hospital. Find out if the doctor is covered by your insurance and if there are extra costs for new-baby care. It's nice to meet and talk with the pediatrician before your partner delivers so you aren't rushed and hassled, as you might be in the hospital. And meeting beforehand allows you the option of choosing someone else if you and your partner do not believe you can form a strong bond and a good relationship with this important healthcare provider.

Exploring child-care options in your area is always a good idea, especially with an infant. You may already have an idea of the cost of child care, but do you know how readily available that care is? You may have to get on a waiting list in some situations. Good infant care is often harder to find because babies require so much more time and energy than older children. You may find that there isn't a lot available in your area, and you may have to sign up fairly early.

All these considerations are important in preparing for baby's arrival. If you are prepared well ahead of time, you can relax knowing you've taken care of some important things.

Chapter Focus

In this chapter, we discuss some of the important preparations you and your partner may want to make before baby's birth. These include choosing the doctor who will care for baby after his or her birth, and selecting the child-care situation that you believe will be best for your baby. These matters are often taken care of before a baby is born so you are prepared when baby finally arrives. In addition, we discuss what things you may want to purchase or to have on hand when baby comes home.

CHOOSING BABY'S DOCTOR

When possible, select the doctor who is going to care for your baby *before* baby's arrival to give you the chance to meet the doctor and to visit his or her practice before you make a final decision. You may want to check out several doctors before you choose the one you and your partner feel the most comfortable with. Make an appointment for an interview 3 to 4 weeks before your baby's due date, in case baby comes early. Topics of discussion might include care in the hospital, whether your partner is planning to breastfeed or if you wish to have your son circumcised.

You have many choices for the type of physician who will care for your baby. They include a pediatrician, a family physician or a general practitioner. A family physician or general practitioner may be the only type of medical doctor available in some areas.

To get suggestions for a referral to a pediatrician, ask friends or family members for the names of doctors they like and trust. Ask your OB/GYN for a reference. If these sources don't provide a name, call your local or county medical society. Check with your insurance provider to see if they have a list of preapproved physicians you *must* use. If you belong to an HMO, contact the patient advocate for information on which pediatricians are accepting new patients.

Once you and your partner choose a physician, call for an appointment. Tell the person you speak with that you are interviewing pediatricians for your soon-to-be-born baby. Some practices hold individual meetings; others have group sessions with several couples. Ask if there is a charge for this initial meeting. Some doctors meet with you for free; others charge a fee for their time.

Below are some questions you might want to ask about the physician. Following the questions are some points to consider after you leave the interview.

Questions to Ask at Your Meeting

Below is a list of questions you may want to think about and then address at the meeting you have with a pediatrician. Some of this information may be important to you; you may not care about other information. One of you can call the physician's office and ask some of these questions of the office staff before your visit, if you have time. You may want to ask other questions when you meet with the doctor to help you create a dialogue about your child's care.

✓ What are your qualifications and training?

✓ What is your availability?

✓ Are your office hours compatible with our schedules?

✓ Do you have weekend office hours?

✓ If we only need medical advice, is there someone we can call and talk with in your office?

✓ Can a sick child be seen the same day?

✓ How can we reach you in case of an emergency or after office hours?

✓ Who responds if you are not available?

✓ Do you have a website or e-mail address?

✓ Do you or your nurse return phone calls the same day?

✓ Do you have X-ray facilities and a laboratory at your office?

Choosing a doctor to care for your little one is a decision you and your partner should make as a couple. Make every effort to attend this visit together. After the visit, you can discuss your reactions to the office staff and the doctor, and decide as a couple whether this is the practice you feel will meet your needs and the needs of your baby.

✓ Are you interested in preventive, developmental and behavioral issues?

✓ How does your practice operate?

✓ Does it comply with our insurance?

✓ Do you have a staff person to file our insurance claims for us?

✓ What is the nearest (to our home) emergency room or urgent-care center we would use?

✓ What happens in special medical situations? To whom do you make referrals?

Other Important Considerations When Selecting a Pediatrician

There are a few issues you can't resolve until you and your partner analyze your feelings after your visit. You may want to examine and to consider how you felt about certain topics you discussed at your meeting, then discuss them together. Below is a list of questions you and your partner might want to address after an initial visit.

✓ Are the doctor's philosophies and attitudes acceptable to us, such as use of antibiotics and other medications, childrearing practices or medically related religious beliefs?

✓ Did he or she seem genuinely interested in our concerns?

✓ Is the doctor going to be available as much as we think we will need him or her to be?

✓ Did the physician appear interested in developing a rapport with our expected child?

✓ Did the physician appear interested in developing a rapport with us?

✓ Is this a person we feel comfortable with and with whom our child will be comfortable?

✓ Did the doctor listen to us?

✓ Did he or she take our concerns seriously?

✓ Do we feel comfortable with this person? Will our child be comfortable with this person?

✓ Is the doctor's age, professional training, board certification (or lack of it), gender, availability, marital status or any other facts about him or her important to us?

CHILD-CARE DECISIONS

Deciding what type of child care is best for your baby can be a challenging task. You and your partner must make many decisions in selecting the type of care you want for your infant. The best way to do that is to know your options before you begin.

In addition to choosing the kind of child care that will suit you as a family, be aware that quality care is in high demand and short supply! Experts advise parents to begin looking for a child-care situation *at least 6 months* before you need it. For some women, that may be the end of the second trimester! If you find a situation you like, sign up as soon as possible; there may be a waiting list. If you find something more suitable later, you can always change your mind.

Before you can determine which type of care you and your partner want, you must examine your needs and the needs of your child. Your options for child care include:

✓ in-your-home care by a family member or by a nonrelative
✓ care in a caregiver's home
✓ a child-care center

In-Home Care

You may choose in-home care, by either a relative or nonrelative. It's fairly easy when someone comes to your home to take care of your child. You don't have to get baby ready before you go in the morning, and you never have to take your child out in bad weather. It also takes less time in the morning and evening if you don't have to drop off or to pick up baby.

When the caregiver is a nonrelative, it can be very expensive to have someone come to your home. You are also hiring someone you do not know to come into your home and tend your child. You must be diligent in asking for references and checking them out thoroughly.

Care in a Caregiver's Home

You and your partner may decide to take your child to someone else's home. A homelike setting may make a child feel comfortable.

However, homes are not regulated in every state, so you must check out each situation very carefully.

You will probably have to pay federal, state and local taxes for your care provider, including Social Security and Medicare taxes. Contact the Internal Revenue Service and your state's Department of Economic Security for further information. If the person works in your home, you may also need to pay Workers' Compensation and unemployment insurance taxes. Be sure you have homeowner's or renter's insurance to cover them while they work in your home.

My Mother-in-Law Said

If a pregnant woman eats the foods she craves, her baby will like those foods, too.

No matter what a pregnant woman eats, it probably won't have much effect on her baby's likes and dislikes of food. Most pregnant woman probably wouldn't want their baby to like some of the weird things they eat, such as pickled herring for breakfast.

Child-Care Centers

A child-care center is an environment in which many children are cared for in a larger setting. Centers vary widely in the facilities and activities they provide, the amount of attention they give each child, group sizes and child-care philosophy.

Some child-care centers do not accept infants. Babies have special needs; be sure the place you choose for your infant can meet those needs.

The Cost of Child Care

It can cost a couple a lot to provide daycare for their child. We're not talking about a situation that is out of the ordinary—we're talking about a regular care situation in your home, someone else's home or in a child-care center. We discuss the cost of child care in Chapter 7; see that discussion for more information.

PREPARING THE NURSERY

You may be surprised at all the baby products you will discover when you begin preparing the nursery. You don't have to buy everything that's out there—be selective, and choose items you think you will use or that other people have told you are really helpful. (A swing is a good example—parents-to-be often overlook a swing as an important piece of equipment. But for some fussy babies, it's a gift from heaven!)

Give some thought about what items you or baby may need. Make a list, and *stick to it!* You or your partner may want to buy every cute

BROWNIE POINTS

Make an effort to keep spending under control. Buy things you *need*, and think twice about things you *want*.

thing you see, but you may be wasting your money if you do. And keep in mind you may receive a lot of baby presents. You'll find that many gifts will be helpful; receiving them as gifts can save you money, too.

You don't always have to buy the most expensive items you find. A high price doesn't necessarily mean a better product. That's why it's important to shop around—for prices *and* information!

You may not think you'll save a lot of money shopping around; however, you can easily spend over $7,500 the first year on baby's necessities and other basics (this includes setting up the nursery with crib, changing table and other items). So take your time and look around—it could be worth your time and effort.

There are a lot of ways to find the best deals for various baby items. Always compare prices of an item at different stores, such as a discount store, a specialty store, an outlet store, a warehouse store and a secondhand store. Check out con-sumer magazines and the Internet, too. Now is the time to check the balance in any special savings ac-count that you created for this pur-pose. The amount you've saved can help you set some spending limits.

IN THE DOGHOUSE

Don't wait until after baby's birth to paint the nursery. Paint fumes aren't healthy for you or the baby to breathe.

We can offer you some other tips, too. Resist impulse buying. Just because you see it and it's cute doesn't mean you have to buy it! Ask other parents what products they've found helpful or necessary. Assess your needs to determine if the products they like can help you. If you don't use something with baby, sell it at a secondhand shop or offer it to someone else. You don't need lots of items cluttering up your house.

You may be surprised how much you can save buying from the least expensive place. Check out the Internet for comparison, if you have a computer. (See the *Resources* section, beginning on page 261.) You may want to try some items before you buy them for comfort and ease of use. For example, if you're thinking of getting a backpack or front carrier, your size can make a difference in how comfortable one type is over another.

Should You Accept Hand-Me-Downs?

You can save quite a bit of money if you use the baby clothes and baby equipment offered by friends and family members. It's a proven fact—babies almost never wear out the clothes they are given before they outgrow them. It can really help your budget if you can borrow a bassinet or use a stroller for a while. You may decide to purchase these items later, or you may only need them for a short time. For example, a baby often grows out of a bassinet in a short time and is more comfortable in a crib.

If you do borrow things, there are some "rules of etiquette" to follow. You and your partner will appear very gracious, and your lender will appreciate your thoughtfulness. Keep in mind the following good manners.

✓ Take good care of everything. There may be times you

Get on a Recall List

You and your partner probably will spend a lot of time deciding what you need for baby and researching the products you're interested in. Wouldn't it be nice to feel secure that every product you buy is safe for baby? That can be a problem because products are occasionally recalled because of design or safety problems.

There are websites on the Internet that can alert you as parents to problems with products and recalls that have been issued. See the *Resources* section for some addresses.

can't, such as when baby spits up on an outfit, but try to keep things clean, in good repair and in good shape.

✓ Find out if the lender wants the item(s) returned and when.

✓ Don't lose track of any items. Make a list of what people lend you, and keep it in a safe place. Return items to the person you borrowed them from.

✓ Write a thank-you note to let the person know you appreciate their generosity.

✓ Do something nice for the lender. Offer to babysit, or make a plate of your famous brownies.

What Equipment Do You Need?

Your baby's nursery can be set up almost anywhere—it may be a separate bedroom, an alcove or an area in your bedroom. Baby can sleep just about anywhere—in a cradle, a bassinet or a crib.

The most essential pieces of equipment you need when you bring baby home are a place for him or her to sleep and a place for diaper changing and dressing. (See the discussion that follows.) If the nursery isn't ready when baby arrives, even a basket or drawer will do for a short time.

Some other items to consider include a comfortable place to sit, such as a rocking chair, a chest of drawers (one that can double as a changing table can save money), a diaper pail, a baby monitor, a small lamp, a mobile, a vaporizer or humidifier, and a smoke detector.

You might consider choosing unfinished furniture. It's usually less expensive, and you can finish it to match the decor in baby's room.

> ### A Word of Caution
>
> Be careful when borrowing or buying someone else's nursery equipment. Some items might not meet current safety standards. If you do borrow something or buy a used item, make sure it meets *all current safety standards*, as established by the federal government. Check out the U.S. Consumer Products Safety Commission website (www.cpsc.gov) or the Juvenile Products Manufacturers Association website (www.jpma.org).

Be creative when it comes to decorations. Use decorative bed sheets and paint to brighten up a room. One wall of wallpaper can provide a theme for the room and add brightness and fun. You don't have to spend a lot of money—baby won't care.

CRIBS AND BASSINETS.   Some parents want baby to sleep in a bassinet in their room for a while. Others put baby in a crib, in his or her own room, from the first day home.

A *bassinet* is a small, portable baby bed that can be used until baby gets too big, then it's time to move to a crib. The bassinet mattress should fit snugly, and sheets must not pull up. A wide base is suggested so it doesn't tip over easily.

A *crib* is more permanent; some cribs are designed to grow with your child and can be converted to a juvenile bed. Before you make a purchase, check out various safety features as established by the Juvenile Products Manufacturers Association (JPMA), the Consumer Product Safety Commission and the American Academy of Pediatrics. See the *Resources* section for contact information.

You'll need some fitted sheets for the crib. Some researchers now believe the crib should be free of *all* items except a fitted sheet and baby—no bumper pads, pillows, comforters or blankets—to help reduce the risk of SIDS (sudden-infant-death syndrome). If baby is chilly, use a zip-up sleeper for warmth. You can use a crib wedge while baby is very young to keep him or her from rolling onto the stomach. (It is now recommended that all babies be put to sleep on their backs to help further reduce the incidence of SIDS.)

Painting Baby's Room

If you're going to paint baby's room before his or her arrival, be sure the paint is nontoxic. If you're unsure what's on the walls now, repaint them with nontoxic paint. It's also a good idea to paint a few weeks in advance of baby's birth, so any paint fumes will have a chance to evaporate. You might want to choose a paint that is low in VOCs (volatile organic compounds). That way you, your partner and baby won't feel any discomfort from the noxious odor of newly applied paint.

BABY CLOTHES.   Baby will need some clothes, but be practical. Most babies can get by just fine with some basic styles for the first year. A few cute outfits are fine, but don't spend your money on them if you don't need to. (You may receive many different clothing items as shower and baby gifts.)

A baby doesn't need as much as you may want to buy. Diapers, T-shirts, gowns that open at the bottom, footed sleepers, socks, bibs, a hat, a warm cover-up, one-piece short- or long-legged "onesies," blankets and towels are the most basic items you need to stock up on. How many of each you need depends on your personal situation.

When choosing diapers, you can choose between disposable diapers and reusable cloth diapers. If you choose cloth diapers, you can wash them yourself or use a diaper service. Or you may choose a combination of cloth and disposable diapers; both types are good in various situations. It's a good idea to have about 8 dozen diapers on hand (order 100 a week for a newborn if you have a diaper service).

In addition to clothes, you'll need some toiletries for baby. A brush and comb, nail clippers or scissors, nasal bulb syringe, an ear-type or rectal thermometer, baby shampoo, diaper-rash ointment, baby oil, baby powder, baby wipes, cotton balls and petroleum jelly can all come in handy when you need them.

BROWNIE POINTS

Wait until *after* your partner's baby showers to buy clothes for your little one. You may not need to spend much money on these items if you receive an entire wardrobe for baby from family and friends. If you do buy things, leave tags on the clothes and save receipts to make it easier to return them if necessary.

DIAPER BAG AND NECESSARY ITEMS.   As parents, you'll learn very quickly that a diaper bag is a lifesaver in many situations. When you're away from home, you can pack along diapers and wipes, extra clothes, bottles or food, pacifiers, toys, a blanket and any other things you'll need.

You can save some money by refraining from buying an expensive designer diaper bag—we've been told by many young fathers and mothers that a sturdy backpack may be one of the best diaper bags around! One of the features they like best? Straps for carrying the bag on their backs instead of in their hands. It provides more freedom and flexibility for handling baby. And an added plus is that you (dad) can wear it or carry it without feeling like you're standing out in a crowd!

CAR SEATS.   The most important piece of baby equipment you can buy is a *car seat*. We suggest a new car seat so you'll know you have the best protection possible when baby takes his or her first ride home from the hospital. Your baby needs to be buckled into his or her car seat *every* time he or she rides in a car—it's the law in all 50 states. The safest place is the middle of the back seat.

Does a baby really need a car seat? Yes! It's the best protection your baby has in case of an accident. Buckle baby up for every ride!

When choosing a car seat for your baby, be certain it meets the safety standards of the JPMA, the Consumer Products Safety Commission and the American Academy of Pediatrics. After you purchase your car seat, and before baby comes home from the hospital, you can have your installation checked by someone who is knowledgeable. Many local police and fire stations will make this check for you and instruct you in proper car-seat installation.

You may choose from an infant-only seat, good until your baby reaches 20 pounds, or a convertible seat, which can be used until your child reaches 40 pounds. With a "combo" type, the car seat is removed and becomes the body of a stroller

---

Making Sure Baby Is Yours

There's an inexpensive new product ($5) that may be available in your area that you may be interested in purchasing. Called the *Birth-Marker*, it's a nontoxic pen that you can use on baby immediately after birth to mark your little bundle of joy with his or her name or some other identifying mark. It's used to prevent accidentally getting the wrong baby in the hospital. The ink comes off with alcohol and shows up on every skin color. See the *Resources* section.

when it is placed in a set of wheels.

If you live in a city and do not have a car, is a car seat necessary? The answer is an emphatic *Yes!* Even if a baby rides in a taxi, he or she should be placed in a safety-restraint system. A choice made by many parents in this situation is a convertible "travel system." It's really three products in one—a car seat, an infant carrier and a stroller. You can use it from birth until baby is a toddler. And it's convenient for you—one product can fulfill many needs.

Turning Baby's Car Seat Around

In the recent past, parents were advised to keep baby in a rear-facing seat position until he or she reached the age of 1 year. Today, some experts advise not turning the car seat around until baby is at least 18 months old. Read the instructions that come with your infant car seat for recommendations.

GETTING YOUR HOUSE READY FOR BABY

In this section, we provide you with some safety tips for making your home safe for your new baby. They can also make your environment safer, too.

Children should live in a smoke-free environment. That means not smoking in the house after baby is born. If you must smoke, do it away from your home. Try to keep your car smoke-free, too. Any time your baby (or your partner, for that matter) inhales secondhand smoke, it exposes him or her to potential harm. Bronchitis, asthma and other respiratory ailments are more common in children when at least one parent smokes.

As we've mentioned earlier in this chapter, check the paint if your home is older. Be sure all painted surfaces are in good condition. If you do any renovations, test the paint for lead content. Call your local health department for information on who can do this for you; you can also buy do-it-yourself test kits at hardware stores. Or call the

IN THE DOGHOUSE

Take care of problems in your home now so the environment will be safe when baby comes home.

National Lead Information Hotline and Clearinghouse at 800-424-LEAD for additional facts.

If you have water damage in your home from a leaking roof, basement flooding or plumbing leaks, you may want to take care of it before baby arrives. Water damage that is ignored can lead to growth of a mold that can cause an infant to develop bleeding lungs, called *pulmonary hemorrhage*. The problem is attributed to a toxic mold that grows on wet wood and paper products. When the mold dries out, its spores can get into the air. If an infant inhales them, they can affect rapidly growing lung cells. This is especially true if baby is under 6 months of age. Dry out wet areas as soon as possible. Throw out any water-soaked items if they don't dry within 24 hours. Replace ceiling tiles that have a dark stain. Clean walls and anything made of wood with a

---

MEMORABLE MOMENTS FROM DR. DAD

Lee and Trish were expecting their baby in October. When the baby decided to come early, in the middle of September, Trish wasn't ready. Following the delivery, she asked Lee to bring some things to the hospital for her, such as a robe, slippers and clothes to wear home. Imagine her surprise when she opened the bag he had packed and found the sexy, lacy negligee and peignoir set he had given her on Valentine's Day the year before. He didn't see any problem with her wearing it while she walked up and down the hospital halls. In addition, he had brought along her prepregnancy designer jeans and a halter top to wear home. For their little boy, he had bought a size 18-month baseball outfit that swallowed him up! Trish broke down and laughed and cried at the same time, then picked up the phone and called her mother to come to her rescue.

mix of one part bleach to four parts water. Take care of any leaks so water damage doesn't recur.

If you have well water and it hasn't been tested, have it tested before baby's birth for *nitrates*. If your baby drinks formula (it's safe to breastfeed, even if mom drinks the water) and the formula is made with water that contains nitrates, baby could develop a life-threatening blood disorder called *methemoglobinemia*. Boiling the water doesn't help—it can actually cause more harm because boiling it *increases* nitrate concentrations. You might want to consider digging a new well or buying bottled water that meets minimum federal safety guidelines to make baby's formula.

10

Childbirth Preparation, and Labor and Delivery

The end is near—at least, the end of pregnancy is near! Quite soon your baby will arrive, and you will all begin your new lives together as a family.

If you are like most men, you don't want to get caught short as the birth of your baby approaches. You and your partner probably want to be prepared for the birth experience and the changes that follow so you'll know what to anticipate. Preparation allows you to deal with the situation more effectively.

To prepare with your partner for the big event, there are quite a few things you might want to address now, others you should know about and still others that you and your partner may want to start thinking about and discussing. This chapter provides you with some of the areas you may want to explore.

Chapter Focus

In this chapter, we look at preparing for, and participating in, the birth of your baby. We discuss childbirth-education classes and examine what they can offer you and your partner. We explore ways to prepare for the birth and advise you what to do when labor begins. As to your experiences in the hospital, we cover everything from pain relief to Cesarean deliveries. After the birth, as a couple you will be faced with new decisions, such as whether to circumcise a baby boy and how your partner will feed baby. We investigate these issues and the actions you might take in each case.

CHILDBIRTH-EDUCATION CLASSES

When you were born, your father may or may not have been an active participant in your birth. Times have changed. Today, many women expect their partner to be at their side, even actively assisting them or participating in the birth process. You may be wondering how you can do this (or even if you *want* to do this)—after all, you may never have had a baby before!

You and your partner can be better prepared for what lies ahead if you take a birth-preparation course. Many couples today take these childbirth-education classes together before their baby is born. In fact, nearly 90% of all first-time expectant parents take some type of class. And they help, too. Studies show that women who take these classes need less medication, have fewer forceps deliveries and feel more positive about birth than women who do not take classes. Having information available beforehand can make you feel more confident and prepared to cope with the birth experience. Before a class begins, you may not believe you will be able to act as your partner's labor coach. After attending classes, you may realize it's an experience you don't want to miss!

The goal of classes is to provide a couple with information so you can both be prepared for what lies ahead. The belief is that if you're better prepared, you'll both be more at ease during labor and delivery. If you're like many men, you may look upon classes as an inconvenience. However, once classes begin, and you start learning how the birth process works and find out what lies ahead, you may find yourself enthusiastic about them.

What to Look for in a Class

Every class has a different style. The list below can help you evaluate whether a childbirth-education class is right for you as a couple.

✓ Class was recommended by our doctor or his or her office staff.

✓ Class uses a philosophy shared by our doctor and childbirth team.

✓ Class begins when we need it, approximately in the 7th month of pregnancy.

✓ Class size is small—no more than 10 or 12 couples—and classroom is large enough to allow all couples the opportunity to practice (on the floor) what they learn in class.

✓ Class includes a tour of the hospital and the labor and delivery areas.

✓ Graduates are enthusiastic. (Locate some, and ask about the class.)

✓ Class is informative, interesting and candid about the birth experience. Pain during labor and delivery is not glossed over or downplayed. The idea of an "ideal birth" is discussed in realistic terms.

✓ Class covers emotional issues and various medical interventions, including induction of labor, Cesarean delivery (C-section), episiotomies and different types of pain-relief methods.

✓ You get to view videos of an actual birth and a Cesarean section, to help you prepare for both.

✓ Information is provided about postbirth issues, such as postpartum distress, circumcision and feeding choices.

✓ Class includes the time and the opportunity to ask questions, practice techniques and talk to parents who have recently given birth.

✓ Classes involving doctors (anesthesiologists, pediatricians) and/or nurses are preferable.

IF YOU CAN'T TAKE A CLASS.   If you cannot find a way to attend classes, check with the hospital or birthing center you have chosen. Try to pick a time that isn't too busy (ask about this when you all); this will give you and your partner the opportunity to ask all your questions. If you show up for your tour and it is extremely busy, reschedule for another time. Taking this tour will help you both feel more comfortable when it's time for your baby to be born.

CHECK OUT THE INSTRUCTOR. The person who teaches the class (nearly all are women) is a very important aspect of the total experience. It can be important for this person to have given birth herself. Some

---

The Language of Labor and Delivery

If you hear terms in classes or at prenatal appointments that you don't understand, check the *Pregnancy-Related Terms for Expecting Couples*, which begins on page 15, for definitions you can understand.

We have found that if a couple is prepared for labor and delivery, the entire experience is more relaxed, even enjoyable. So if your partner brings up the subject of attending childbirth-education classes together, be open to the experience!

Most childbirth-education classes run for about 6 weeks—you and your partner attend one class each week. However, if you can't find the time in your schedules to attend this many classes, consider an all-day class or a weekend class. A short class is better than no class!

If this is too much to handle at one time, think about private, individualized sessions in your home. An instructor comes to you, when you are free; classes can be as long or as short as your schedules permit.

instructors are medically trained, such as a labor-and-delivery nurse; others have no medical training at all. Check out instructor qualifications.

Major Childbirth Philosophies

You and your partner may be wondering if one type of delivery method covered in childbirth-education classes is better than another. Any method can be the right one for you as a couple, but it's best for you both to agree on one method. It is also important to discuss this with the doctor for his or her input. If your partner chooses a method that greatly involves you, and you aren't willing or able to provide that level of involvement, it could lead to disappointment and anxiety.

Childbirth-preparation methods are usually divided among three major philosophies—Lamaze, Bradley and Grantly Dick-Read. Each philosophy offers its own techniques and methods. In addition, other organizations certify childbirth educators, including the Association of Labor Assistants and Childbirth Educators (ALACE), Birth Works, Inc. and the International Childbirth Education Association (ICEA).

Lamaze is the oldest technique of childbirth preparation; about 25% of all pregnant women in America take these courses. Through training, it conditions mothers to replace unproductive laboring efforts with effective ones because the Lamaze philosophy is that birth is a normal, natural, healthy process. It emphasizes relaxation and breathing as ways to ease pain during labor and delivery. In recent years, partners have been included in Lamaze classes.

Robert Bradley, M.D., believed fathers should help in childbearing—his belief is one reason there are so many men participating in births today. *Bradley* classes teach relaxation and inward focus; many types of relaxation are used. Strong emphasis is put on relaxation and deep abdominal breathing to make labor more comfortable. Classes often begin when pregnancy is confirmed and continue until after the birth. Women in Bradley classes typically have decided they do not want to use any type of medication for labor-pain relief.

BROWNIE POINTS

Look at childbirth-education classes as a way to help you prepare, as a couple, for the birth experience. Information and techniques to help you deal with this unfamiliar situation can be very beneficial.

Grantly Dick-Read is a method that attempts to break the fear–tension–pain cycle of labor and delivery through training in and practice of particular techniques. These classes were the first to include fathers in the birth experience.

The *Association of Labor Assistants and Childbirth Educators (ALACE)* began in the 1970s as a home-birth preparation class. However, today classes teach relaxation and coping methods to help a woman through the pain and discomfort of giving birth, wherever she delivers.

Birth Works, Inc. is an organization whose goal is to help women undergo more positive birth experiences. Members attempt to do this by helping to teach women to trust more in their own instincts about their bodies.

The *International Childbirth Education Association (ICEA)* doesn't advocate any particular birth philosophy or take a stand regarding pain relief during birth. They provide information to help a couple make choices based on their knowledge of alternatives.

Choosing Your Class

Begin looking into classes that are offered in your area about halfway through the second trimester—around 20 weeks of pregnancy is a good point to start. Ask your doctor or the office nurse to recommend classes in your area; he or she should be pretty familiar with what is offered. Friends can also be good sources, or look in the yellow pages under *Childbirth Education*. You may have to sign up early. Classes should start by the beginning of the third trimester (about 27 weeks). Try to finish the classes at least a few weeks before the due date.

> Learning what you need to know to have a positive birth experience is fine, but it's important to practice what you learn in your classes. Follow the guidelines and instructions you learn in your classes. Aim for at least 20 minutes of practice a day. If you can't spare that much time, four 30-minute sessions each week should be beneficial. If you don't practice what you learn, you won't be able to put it into action when you need to.

Childbirth classes may be offered in many settings, such as community centers, universities or churches. Most hospitals that deliver babies offer prenatal classes on site. They are often taught by labor-and-delivery nurses or by a midwife.

The cost of classes can range from $50 to over $300 (for private instruction). Some insurance companies and a few HMOs offer partial or full reimbursement for class fees. Ask the human resources person at work or call your insurance company to see if classes are covered.

WILL YOU BE THE LABOR COACH?

Are you looking forward to being an important part of your baby's birth? If you are, you're not alone. Many men today take an active role in the birth process and enjoy their participation.

Sharing the birth of your child with your partner can have an effect neither of you may see for a while. Studies show that couples who share this moving experience grow closer emotionally and become more intimate in the months that follow. In addition, your presence may reassure your partner and give her confidence that everything will be OK. Research indicates that when a woman is overly fearful or anxious, it can interfere with the birth process. Your presence may help relax your partner and make her feel confident she can do this important job.

What If I Can't Do It?

It's not unusual for a man to have some fear or dread about participating in the birth. You may feel queasy at the thought of being in the delivery room or fear you'll pass out at the sight of a lot of blood. Or you may believe it will be too difficult to see your partner in pain and not be able to do much about it. Society puts a lot of pressure on you with its expectation that you take on a role that could make you very uncomfortable. You need to decide what you can do, and discuss it with your partner.

> **IN THE DOGHOUSE**
>
> If you're going to participate in labor and delivery, take your role seriously. Your partner and everyone else at the delivery will appreciate it; so will you.

If you do not believe you will be able to act as your partner's labor coach, especially after your childbirth-education classes, be honest with her. Let her know what you're willing to do—from sitting in the waiting room to participating in a limited way, such as standing next to her and holding her hand. Your frankness will serve you better than pretending you can do something then not being able to follow through with it.

What Does the Labor Coach Do?

A good labor coach can help make the birth experience positive and rewarding. The key lies in establishing good communication between the two of you. Ask your partner to tell you what she wants you to do once

> Although your partner is the one who is in labor, your experience can also be very intense. If you find you need support during your partner's labor, call a close friend or relative to be there for you. The important thing to remember is to try to stay relaxed during this time.

her contractions begin. Knowing what is expected of you helps you provide her with what she needs and wants. But be aware that you'll both need to be flexible. Labor and delivery are an adventure; there are lots of unknowns. During labor, a situation can quickly change, and a new plan may need to be put into action. As much as we would like to plan labor and delivery, it isn't possible. Anticipate the unexpected, then deal with it together.

LABOR COACH'S DOS AND DON'TS.   Below is a list of some labor coach dos and don'ts. Read them over so you will be familiar with what is expected of you. You'll also know what *not* to do! Add to the list anything else you learned in your childbirth-education classes.

✓ Do be your partner's advocate. Inform the hospital staff when she is in pain or when labor activity changes. Keep out unwanted visitors. Ask for items your partner needs.

✓ Do help with timing contractions.

✓ Do assist your partner in her breathing techniques. Know which technique is appropriate for different stages of labor.

✓ Do listen to the labor nurse; she may offer excellent advice, based on her experience.

✓ Do remain flexible. Things can quickly change, and plans may also need to change.

✓ Do offer ice chips or a damp washcloth to your partner if she becomes dehydrated.

✓ Do try to distract your partner when the time seems right.

✓ Do whatever you can to make your partner more comfortable. Ask her what she wants.

✓ Do offer to massage your partner's sore back or aching muscles.

✓ Do let your partner make major decisions about aspects of the birth, such as whether she needs pain medication.

✓ Do take a break if you need it; be sure to let the nurse know where you are going and when you'll return.

✓ Do make a big deal of the birth of your baby by bringing your partner flowers or a special treat after baby arrives. Celebrate!

✓ Do whatever you can to make the experience the best it can be for both of you.

✓ Don't wait too long before you take your partner to the hospital.

✓ Don't take things personally. If your partner gets touchy or seems angry with you, ignore it.

✓ Don't stay in the labor or delivery room if it's too much for you. The staff can care for only one patient (your laboring partner) at a time.

✓ Don't leave the labor room to make phone calls for work; don't take work into the labor room.

✓ Don't leave without letting someone know where you are going.

✓ Don't be too attentive. Give your partner the attention she wants; leave her alone when she doesn't want it.

✓ Don't take pictures if your partner asks you not to.

Choosing Another Labor Coach
Although it is nice for your partner to have you act as her labor coach, it's not mandatory. She can choose a friend or family member to act as her coach. Don't be offended if she asks someone else.

Women who are professionally trained to assist a woman in labor are called *doulas* (see the discussion below); the mom-to-be may choose one to help her. Sometimes the pregnant woman will choose someone who used the same childbirth practice, such as the Lamaze, the Bradley or the Grantly-Dick Read method, for a recent birth.

Your Participation, If You're Not the Labor Coach
Even if you and your partner agree that it's OK to have someone else serve as her labor coach, you can still be involved in the birth experience without having to be involved in the actual labor and birth processes. You can be in the delivery room and can help in many ways, such as:

✓ timing your partner's contractions so you are both aware of labor's progress

✓ encouraging and reassuring the mom-to-be during labor

✓ helping create a mood in the labor room

✓ protecting privacy for both of you, controlling who visits and when, and overseeing telephone calls

✓ reporting to family members how labor is progressing

✓ playing music, reading or distracting your partner in some other way

✓ cutting the baby's umbilical cord after the birth

You don't have to take an active part in the labor process to support your partner emotionally. Just being together can help you both during this wondrous time. Sharing in the joy of your baby's birth can begin your bonding experience as a family.

What Is a Doula?

Your partner may choose a doula to assist her during birth. A *doula* is a woman who is trained to provide support and assistance to a

---

Questions to Ask a Prospective Doula

If your partner is considering a doula to assist her during labor and delivery, it's a good idea to interview a few before you choose one. Some questions you, as a couple, may want to ask and some perceptions you might want to analyze after your interview are listed below.

• What are your qualifications and training? Are you certified? By which organization?

• Have you had a baby yourself? What childbirth method did you use?

• What is your childbirth philosophy?

• Are you familiar with the method we have chosen (if you have a particular method you want to use)?

• What kind of plan would you use to help us through our labor?

• How available are you to answer our questions before the birth?

• How often will we meet before the birth?

• How do we contact you when labor begins?

• What happens if you aren't available when we go into labor?

• Are you experienced in helping a new mom with breastfeeding? How available are you after the birth to help with this and other postpartum problems?

• What is your fee?

Perceptions include how easy the doula is to talk to and to communicate with. Did she listen well and answer your questions? Did you feel comfortable with her?

If you don't hit it off with one doula, try another!

woman during labor and delivery of her baby. The doula remains with the woman from the onset of labor until her baby is born.

A doula is different from a midwife because a doula does not deliver babies. Her strength comes in the form of physical and emotional support to a woman during labor and delivery. This ranges from giving a laboring woman a massage to helping the woman focus on her breathing. A doula may even be able to help the new mother begin breastfeeding her baby.

The real strength of a doula is to provide support to a woman who has chosen to have a drug-free labor and delivery. If your partner has decided she wants anesthesia, no matter what, a doula may not be a wise choice.

Although a doula's primary function is to provide support to the expectant mother during labor, she often assists the labor coach. She does not displace a labor coach; she works with him or her. However, in some situations, a doula may *serve* as the labor coach.

The services of a doula may be expensive and can range from $250 to $1,500. This covers labor and one or more prenatal visits.

If you and your partner choose to have a doula present during labor and the birth, talk to your doctor about your decision. He or she may find her presence intrusive and veto the idea. Or the doctor may be able to give you the name of someone he or she often works with.

AS THE BIRTH DATE APPROACHES

Now that the delivery date is drawing near, it's time to talk with your partner about how you will stay in touch with each other. Some people rent personal pagers for the last few weeks. (Some hospitals or HMOs supply pagers for expectant couples.) With cellular phones so readily available now, staying in touch is even easier. If you don't have a cell phone, you may be able to borrow one from a friend or family member. Arrange for a backup support person, in case you cannot be with your partner or your partner needs someone else to take her to the hospital.

Before Labor Begins

By now, you and your partner may be impatient for your baby's birth. But you may be unsure when labor actually begins. When the day finally comes, you need to be aware of the signs that indicate labor has started. Signs you and your partner may notice include:

✓ increase of Braxton-Hicks contractions

✓ baby "drops" lower into your partner's pelvis

✓ your partner experiences weight loss or a break in weight gain

✓ she feels increased pressure in the pelvis and rectum

✓ there are changes in her vaginal discharge

✓ she has diarrhea

Preparing for the Birth

Your partner may already have her hospital bag packed and ready to go. Do you have one ready for yourself? It's a good idea to pack a backpack or small bag with some essentials to help you during the birth. You might bring the following for yourself:

✓ comfortable shoes

✓ a change of clothes

✓ a watch with a second hand

✓ toiletries, such as deodorant, toothbrush, toothpaste

✓ powder for massaging your partner during labor

✓ a small paint roller or tennis ball for giving your partner a low-back massage during labor

✓ tapes or CDs and a player, or a radio to play during labor

✓ camera and film, or a videocamera (*only* if you both agree to recording the birth)

✓ list of telephone numbers, change or a prepaid calling card or a long-distance calling card

✓ change for telephones and vending machines

✓ nonperishable snacks and a filled water bottle

✓ reading material

If Your Partner's Water Breaks

Inside your partner's uterus, the baby is surrounded by amniotic fluid. As labor begins, the membranes that surround the baby and hold the fluid ("waters") may break, and fluid leaks from the vagina. When the bag of waters breaks, often there is a gush of fluid, followed by slow leaking. Or your partner may just feel a slow leaking, without the gush of fluid.

Not every woman's water breaks before she goes into labor. Often the physician must rupture the membranes during labor. If your partner believes her water has broken, call the doctor immediately. You may be advised to take her to the hospital.

Occasionally the bag of waters breaks before baby is ready to be born. If your partner is not near term, your doctor may ask her to come to the office for an examination. Be sure you or someone else can take her to this appointment because when membranes rupture, things can happen quickly.

If your baby is not ready to be born yet, the doctor will want to confirm that your partner's water has broken and to take measures to prevent infection. The risk of infection increases when a woman's water breaks.

MEMORABLE MOMENTS FROM DR. DAD

When I got to the hospital to deliver their baby, Heather told me about rousing Chris for the journey. She had awakened during the night with contractions, but she didn't want to waken Chris in case they went away like they had before. They had gone to the hospital the night before, only to find out it was false labor, so Heather decided to let Chris sleep while she timed her contractions. When the contractions got to be about 3 minutes apart, she woke Chris and told him it was time to go to the hospital—this was the real thing. He sleepily asked how often she was having contractions. She said they were 3 minutes apart. Not quite awake, he rolled over in bed, telling her to wake him when the contractions were 5 minutes apart! Turning the lights on and shaking him awake, she exclaimed the contractions weren't going to get farther apart. She was in labor, and it was time to go to the hospital now!

TIMING CONTRACTIONS.   It's important for your doctor to know how often contractions occur and how long each one lasts. By knowing this, he or she can help you decide if it's time to go to the hospital. Contractions are timed to see how long a contraction lasts and how often contractions occur. Ask your doctor how he or she prefers you to time them. There are two ways to do it.

Method 1. Start timing when the contraction starts, and time it until the next contraction starts. (This is the most common method.)

Method 2. Start timing when the contraction ends, and note how long it is until the next contraction starts.

GOING TO THE HOSPITAL

You and your partner may want to preregister at the hospital a few weeks before your due date. It will save time checking in, and it may help reduce stress. Preregister with forms you receive from the doctor's office or from the hospital. Even if you don't actually take them to the hospital before labor begins, it's a good idea to fill out the forms early. If you wait until your partner is in labor, you may be in a hurry and concerned with other things.

Be sure you take your partner's insurance card or insurance information with you—have it readily at hand. It's also helpful to know your partner's blood type and Rh-factor, your doctor's name, your pediatrician's name and the due date.

Ask your doctor how you should prepare to go to the hospital; he or she may have specific instructions for you. You might want to ask the following questions.

✓ When should we go to the hospital once my partner is in labor?

✓ Should we call you before we leave for the hospital?

✓ How can we reach you after regular office hours?

✓ Are there any particular instructions for us to follow during early labor?

✓ Where do we go—to the emergency room or the labor-and-delivery department?

The Labor Check

When you take your partner to the hospital, you may both be sent home! This happens if labor hasn't really started or if it is early labor. When you arrive at the hospital, your partner will be evaluated for signs of labor. This is sometimes called a *labor check*.

If your partner is sent home, don't get frustrated, upset or mad. Understand that to determine if a woman is in labor she must often be seen and evaluated at the hospital. This is something that can't be determined over the phone!

The people who evaluate your partner know you want to get on with the birth process and that you don't want to go home. However, if your partner isn't in true labor (see the box below for a comparison of true and false labor), it *is* best to go home. If this happens to you, be supportive of your partner. Try to help her understand that you'll come back when the time is right!

TRUE LABOR OR FALSE LABOR?

Considerations	True Labor	False Labor
Contractions	Regular	Irregular
Time between contractions	Gets closer together	Does not get closer together
Contraction intensity	Increases	Doesn't change
Location of contractions	Entire abdomen or back	Various locations
Effect of anesthetic or pain relievers	Will not stop labor	Sedation may alter frequency or stop contractions
Cervical change	Progressive cervical change (effacement and dilatation)	No cervical change

After Your Partner Is Admitted to the Hospital

When your partner is admitted to labor and delivery (or a birthing center), many things happen. She is checked to see how much her cervix has dilated. A brief pregnancy history is taken. Vital signs, including blood pressure, pulse, temperature and baby's heart rate, are noted. Your partner may receive an enema, or an intravenous drip may be started; blood will probably be drawn. Your partner may have an epidural put in place, if she requests one.

A copy of the mother-to-be's office chart is usually kept on record; it contains basic information about your partner's health and pregnancy. An initial pelvic exam is performed to help determine what stage of labor she is in and to use as a reference point for future exams during labor. This exam and the vital signs are performed by a labor-and-delivery nurse (the nurse can be male or female). Only in unusual situations, such as in an emergency, will your doctor do this initial exam. In fact, it may be quite awhile before you see your doctor, but rest assured the nurses are in close telephone contact with him or her. In many labors, the doctor does not arrive until close to delivery.

> During the time your partner is getting settled in, you may want to alert family members that you're at the hospital. Use the time to call your employer and your partner's employer to let them know that labor has begun. Do these things at this time so you don't have to leave your partner when she needs you later.

If your partner has decided to have an epidural or if it looks as if labor will last quite awhile, an I.V. will be started. Your partner can still walk around. She will probably not be allowed to have more than ice chips or small sips of water. During this time, you may be alone with your partner, with nurses coming into the room to perform various tasks, then leaving. In most instances, a monitoring belt is placed on the mother-to-be's abdomen to record her contractions and the baby's heartbeat. The monitoring record can be seen in the room and also by nurses at the nursing station.

Blood pressure is taken at regular intervals, and pelvic exams are performed to follow labor's progress. In most places, the doctor is notified upon your admission to labor and delivery; he or she is then called at regular intervals as labor progresses. Your doctor will also be called if any problem arises.

In some cases, when you get to the hospital you will learn your doctor is not available and someone else will deliver your baby. If your doctor believes he or she might be out of town when your baby is born, ask to meet doctors that "cover" when your doctor is unavailable. Although your physician would like to be there for the birth of your baby, sometimes it is not possible.

WAYS YOUR PARTNER CAN COPE WITH LABOR AND CHILDBIRTH PAIN

Most first-time mothers have no idea how painful labor and delivery might be. We believe it's important to state the truth—childbirth is nearly always accompanied by pain. Pain varies among women, from a little to a lot, and it can also vary from one delivery to the next. Research shows that the *expectation* of pain can, in itself, evoke fear and anxiety. The best way to deal with pain is to become informed about it.

Some women believe they shouldn't ask for pain relief during labor. They may believe the baby will be harmed by the medication they take. Other women believe they'll deprive themselves of the "complete birth experience." Still others are concerned about cost and believe they can't afford an epidural if their insurance doesn't cover it. Don't put that kind of pressure on your partner, and don't let anyone else do it either.

You and your partner will probably learn about pain and pain relief through various channels. Childbirth-education classes are a source of information; however, some instructors do not address the pain issue sufficiently. They may gloss over how much pain a woman may experience. In classes, you may learn about pain-relief methods that don't require medication, such as breathing methods and relaxation techniques. Some classes include information about epidurals and even invite an anesthesiologist to describe the procedure in one of the classes.

If you and your partner are concerned about how she will deal with pain during labor and delivery, talk to your doctor about pain-relief methods. Using medication for pain relief is usually a personal choice, not a medical decision.

Encourage your partner to keep an open mind about using pain-relief medication during labor. Her labor may be harder (or easier) than anticipated, and she may have a greater or lesser need for pain relief. She can usually change her mind if she needs to or wants to. Be supportive of her choice. You may have a hard time relating to the pain involved in labor and delivery.

Pain Relief without Medication

Some women prefer to try different laboring positions, massage, breathing patterns, relaxation techniques or hypnotherapy to relieve pain. Breathing patterns and relaxation techniques are usually learned in a childbirth-education class.

BROWNIE POINTS

Take the time to practice breathing and relaxation techniques *before* baby's birth so you'll be able to use them effectively. Remember—practice makes perfect!

Different laboring positions and massage enable a woman and her labor coach to work together during labor to find relief. Some women say using these methods brought them closer to their partner and made the birth experience a more joyful one for both of them.

MASSAGE FOR RELIEF.   Massage is one way to help a woman feel better during labor. The touching and caressing of massage can help her relax. One study showed that women who were massaged for 20 minutes every hour during active labor felt less anxiety and less pain.

Massaging the head, neck, back and feet can offer comfort and relaxation. The person doing the massage should pay close attention to the woman's responses to determine correct pressure.

Different types of massage affect a woman in various ways. You and your partner may want to practice the two types of massage described below before labor begins so you're familiar with both.

> ### My Mother-in-Law Said
>
> *With every woman's first baby, labor is very long and delivery is extremely painful.*
>
> This is simply not true. We know of many first-time mothers who had short labors, those whose deliveries were relatively pain-free and even some lucky women who had their first babies in a relatively short time, with little pain!

Effleurage is light, gentle fingertip massage over the abdomen and upper thighs; it is used during early labor. Stroking is light, but doesn't tickle, and fingertips never leave the skin. Start with hands on either side of the navel. Move the hands upward and outward, and come back down to the pubic area. Move the hands back up to the navel. Massage may extend down the thighs. It can also be done as a crosswise motion, around fetal-monitor belts (if present). Move fingers across the abdomen from one side to the other, between the belts.

Counterpressure massage is excellent for relieving the pain of back labor. Place the heel of the hand or the flat part of the fist (you can also use a tennis ball) against the tailbone. Apply firm pressure in a small, circular motion.

Analgesics and Anesthetics

There are many different types of pain relief. Analgesia and anesthesia include a variety of methods. Knowing about each type may help you and your partner make decisions about which one is right for her.

ANALGESIA. *Analgesia* decreases the pain of labor, but the woman remains conscious. It provides pain relief but can make a woman drowsy, restless or nauseous. It may slow the baby's reflexes and breathing, so medication is usually given only during early and middle parts of labor. Examples of analgesia are Demerol (meperidine hydrochloride) and morphine.

GENERAL ANESTHESIA.   A woman is completely unconscious under *general anesthesia,* so it is used only for some Cesarean deliveries and emergency vaginal deliveries. The baby is also anesthetized and needs to be resuscitated after delivery. General anesthesia is not used very often for childbirth today. Its advantage is that it can be administered quickly in an emergency.

LOCAL ANESTHESIA.   *Local anesthesia* affects a small area and is useful for an episiotomy and episiotomy repair. An *episiotomy* is a surgical incision in the area between the vagina and the rectum, that is made to avoid tearing or lacerating the vaginal opening or rectum during the birth. It rarely affects the baby and usually has few lingering effects.

REGIONAL ANESTHESIA.   *Regional anesthesia* affects a larger body area than local anesthesia. The three most common types of regional anesthesia are pudendal block, spinal block and epidural block.

A *pudendal block* is medication injected into the pudendal nerve area in the vagina to relieve pain in the vaginal area, the perineum and the rectum. The woman is conscious, and side effects are rare. Pudendal block is considered one of the safest forms of pain relief; however, it does not relieve uterine pain (the pain of contractions).

With a *spinal block,* medication is injected into spinal fluid in the lower back and numbs the lower part of the body. The woman remains conscious. This is administered only once during labor, so it is often used just before delivery or for a Cesarean section. It works quickly and is an effective pain inhibitor.

For an *epidural block,* a tube is inserted into a space outside the spinal column in the lower back. It is given when labor is very active, the cervix is dilating and pain is increasing. The procedure requires using a needle to insert a small tube or catheter between two vertebrae located in the lower back. Medication is administered through the tube for pain relief, and the woman remains conscious during delivery. The tube remains in place until after the birth so medication can be readministered as necessary. An epidural relieves painful uterine contractions and pain in the vagina and rectum as the baby passes through the birth canal. It is also used to deal with episiotomy pain. A woman still feels pressure sensations so she is able to push during vaginal delivery. However, an epidural may make it harder to push, so vacuum extraction or forceps may be necessary during delivery.

THE BABY'S BIRTH POSITION

Most babies enter the birth canal head first, which is the best position for labor and delivery. However, some babies enter the birth canal in other positions.

A *breech position* means the baby is not in a head-down position; its legs or buttocks come into the birth canal first. If your baby is breech when it is time to deliver, your doctor may try to turn the baby or your partner may require a Cesarean delivery.

For a long time, breech deliveries were performed vaginally. Then it was believed the safest delivery method was a C-section; many doctors still prefer to do a Cesarean for a breech presentation. However, some physicians believe a woman can deliver a breech baby without difficulty if the situation is right. If this situation occurs, your doctor will discuss it with both of you.

DELIVERY OF YOUR BABY

Vaginal Delivery of Your Baby
After your partner has labored through the first stage, she is ready to deliver your baby. You will both finally meet your child, for whom you have waited for so long.

STAGES OF LABOR

Stage 1—Early Phase

What's happening
- Cervix opens and thins out due to uterine contractions
- Cervix dilates to about 2cm
- This phase can last 1 to 10 hours

Mother is experiencing
- Membranes may rupture, accompanied by gush or trickle of amniotic fluid from vagina
- Pinkish discharge may appear ("bloody show")
- Mild contractions begin at 15- to 20-minute intervals; they last about 1 minute
- Contractions become closer together and more regular

What mother or labor coach can do
- Mother should not eat or drink anything once labor begins
- Mother may be able to stay at home, if she is at term
- Begin using relaxation and breathing techniques learned in childbirth class
- If water has broken, if labor is preterm, if there is intense pain, if pain is constant or there is bright red blood, contact doctor immediately!

Stage 1—Active Phase

What's happening
- Cervix dilates from about 2 to 10cm
- Cervix continues to thin out
- This phase can last 20 minutes to 2 hours

Mother is experiencing
- Contractions become more intense
- Contractions come closer together
- Contractions are about 3 minutes apart and last about 45 seconds to 1 minute

What mother and labor coach can do
- Keep practicing relaxation and breathing techniques
- An epidural can be administered during this phase

Stage 1—Transition Phase

What's happening
- Stage 1 begins to change to Stage 2
- Cervix is dilated to 10cm
- Cervix continues to thin out
- This phase can last a few minutes to 2 hours

Mother is experiencing
- Contractions are 2 to 3 minutes apart and last about 1 minute
- Mother may feel strong urge to push; she shouldn't push until cervix is completely dilated
- Mother may be moved to delivery room if she is not in a birthing room

What mother and labor coach can do
- Relaxation and breathing techniques help counteract mother's urge to push

Stage 2—Baby Is Born

What's happening
- Cervix is completely dilated
- Baby continues to descend into the birth canal
- As mother pushes, baby is delivered
- Doctor or nurse suctions baby's nose and mouth, and clamps umbilical cord
- This stage can last a few minutes to a few hours (pushing the baby can last a long time)

Mother is experiencing
- Contractions occur at 2- to 5-minute intervals and last from 60 to 90 seconds
- With an epidural, mother may find it harder to push
- An episiotomy may be done to prevent tearing vaginal tissues as baby is born

What mother and labor coach can do
- Mother will begin to push with each contraction after cervix dilates completely
- Mother may be given analgesic or local anesthetic
- Mother must listen to doctor or nurse when baby is being delivered; doctor or nurse will tell mother when to push
- As mother pushes, she may be able to watch baby being born, if mirror is available

Stage 3—The Placenta Is Delivered

What's happening
- Placenta is delivered
- Doctor examines placenta to make sure all of it has been delivered
- Doctor repairs episiotomy
- This stage can last a few minutes to an hour

Mother is experiencing
- Contractions may occur closer together but be less painful

What mother and labor coach can do
- Meet and hold the baby
- Mother may need to push to expel the placenta
- Mother may be able to hold baby while the doctor repairs episiotomy
- Nurse will rub or massage the uterus through the abdomen to help it contract and to control bleeding (during the next few days, the uterus will continue to contract to control bleeding)

The actual delivery of the baby and placenta (not including the laboring process) in stage 2 takes from a few minutes to an hour or more. See the boxes on pages 228–230 describing the *Stages of Labor.*

Once full dilatation of the cervix is reached (10cm), pushing begins. Pushing can take 1 to 2 hours (first or second baby) to a few minutes (an experienced mom). Delivery of the baby, placenta and repair of the episiotomy usually takes 20 to 30 minutes.

Following delivery, the baby and your partner are evaluated. During this time, you finally get to see and to hold your baby, and your partner can even feed the baby. The part that takes the longest may not be the birth of the baby; stitching closed the various skin and muscle layers after baby is born may take the greatest amount of time.

Depending on whether your partner delivers in a hospital or birthing center, she may deliver in the same room she has been laboring in (often called *LDRP* for labor, delivery, recovery and postpartum). She may be moved to a delivery room nearby. After the birth, she will go to recovery for a short time, then move to a hospital room until she's ready to go home.

Cesarean Delivery

In some cases, complications may occur during labor; these complications may require a Cesarean delivery, also called a *C-section.* With a Cesarean section, the baby is delivered through an incision made in the mother's abdominal wall and uterus. While there are many reasons for doing a C-section, the main goal is the same as a vaginal delivery—to deliver a healthy baby and to ensure the health of the mother.

> In most situations in which a C-section is required, you'll be able to stay with your partner until the procedure is complete. Ask the doctor about it if you want to stay. And ask what is involved, so you can decide whether you want to remain in the delivery room or wait outside.

A couple often wants to know in advance if they will need a Cesarean delivery. A doctor doesn't usually know the answer to this question before labor begins, unless the woman has had a previous C-section, the baby is breech or there are other complications. We usually have to wait for labor contractions to begin before we can tell if the baby is stressed by them or if the baby fits through the birth canal.

A Cesarean delivery is major surgery and carries with it certain risks. If your partner has a C-section, she will probably have to stay in the hospital for a couple of extra days. Recovery is slower with a Cesarean than with a vaginal delivery. Full recovery normally takes 4 to 6 weeks.

It's a good idea for you and your partner to discuss Cesarean delivery with your doctor several weeks before the due date. Ask why he or she would do a C-section. Express your wishes and concerns, as a couple, in regards to having a Cesarean delivery.

EMERGENCY DELIVERY ALONE

1. Call 911 for help.

2. Call a neighbor, family member or friend.

3. Try not to push or to bear down.

4. Spread out towels and blankets in a comfortable place.

5. If the baby comes before help arrives, try to use your hands to ease the baby out while you gently push.

6. Wrap the baby in a clean blanket or clean towels; hold it close to your body to keep it warm.

7. Use a clean cloth to remove mucus from the baby's mouth.

8. Do not pull on the umbilical cord to deliver the placenta.

9. If the placenta delivers on its own, save it.

10. You don't need to cut the cord.

11. Keep yourself and baby warm until medical help arrives.

EMERGENCY DELIVERY AT HOME

1. Call 911 for help.

2. Call a neighbor, family member or friend (have phone numbers available).

3. Encourage the woman *not* to push or to bear down.

4. Use blankets and towels to make the woman as comfortable as possible.

5. If there is time, wash the woman's vaginal and rectal areas with soap and water.

6. When the baby's head delivers, encourage the woman to pant or blow, and to concentrate on *not* pushing.

7. Try to ease the baby's head out with gentle pressure. Do not pull on the head.

8. After the head is delivered, gently push down on the head and push a little to deliver the shoulders.

9. As one shoulder delivers, lift the head up, delivering the other shoulder. The rest of the baby will quickly follow.

10. Wrap the baby in a clean blanket or towel.

11. Use a clean cloth or tissue to remove mucus from the baby's mouth.

12. Do not pull on the umbilical cord to deliver the placenta—it is not necessary.

13. If the placenta delivers on its own, wrap it in a towel or clean newspapers and save it.

14. You don't need to cut the cord.

15. Keep the placenta at the level of the baby or above the baby.

16. Keep both mother and baby warm with towels or blankets until medical help arrives.

EMERGENCY DELIVERY
ON THE WAY TO THE HOSPITAL

1. Stop the car.

2. Try to get help, if you have a cellular phone or CB radio.

3. Put on your flashing hazard lights.

4. Place the woman in the backseat, with a towel or blanket under her.

5. Encourage the woman not to push or to bear down.

6. When the baby's head delivers, encourage the woman to pant or blow, and to concentrate on *not* pushing.

7. Try to ease the baby's head out with gentle pressure. Do not pull on the head.

8. After the head is delivered, gently push down on the head and push a little to deliver the shoulders.

9. As one shoulder delivers, lift the head up, delivering the other shoulder. The rest of the baby will quickly follow.

10. Wrap the baby in a clean blanket or towel. Use clean newspapers if nothing else is available.

11. Use a clean cloth or tissue to remove mucus from the baby's mouth.

12. Do not pull on the umbilical cord to deliver the placenta—it is not necessary.

13. If the placenta delivers on its own, wrap it in a towel or clean newspapers and save it.

14. You don't need to cut the cord.

15. Keep the placenta at the level of the baby or above the baby.

16. Keep both mother and baby warm until you can get them to the hospital or medical help arrives.

AFTER YOUR BABY IS BORN

Things happen quickly once baby emerges into the world. First, baby's mouth and throat are suctioned. Then the doctor clamps and cuts the umbilical cord (or you may cut the cord). If you want to cut the umbilical cord after the baby is delivered, discuss it with your doctor *before* labor. What you may be allowed to do varies in certain situations and from place to place.

The baby is then wrapped in clean blankets and may be placed on your partner's abdomen. Apgar scores are recorded at 1 minute and 5 minutes after birth. An identification band is placed on baby's wrist or ankle. Usually a brief physical exam or an assessment is done right after delivery. The baby receives drops in its eyes to prevent infection and is given a vitamin K shot to prevent bleeding. You will be asked if you want your baby to receive the hepatitis vaccine. Discuss this with your doctor before the birth; the vaccine protects your baby against hepatitis in the future.

When the initial evaluation is complete, baby is returned to you and your partner. Later, baby is placed in a heated bassinet for a period of time.

THE CIRCUMCISION DECISION

If you have a son, you will have an additional decision to make—whether he will be circumcised. When a baby boy is *circumcised,* the skin that covers the end of his penis is removed. This may be done as a surgical procedure, or a clamping device may be used to remove the foreskin. It is usually performed at the hospital; however if you are Jewish or Muslim, it may be done as part of a religious ceremony, outside of the hospital.

Today, about 65% of all male babies are circumcised—in the 1970s, that number was as high as 80%. It is not unusual now for a couple to decide *not* to have their son circumcised. Whatever decision is made, you and your partner should make it together. Work this out *before* baby is born, so you both understand the issue and agree on what steps to take after your baby's birth.

Other than for religious purposes, infant boys are circumcised for two reasons. The main reason many couples give is that they don't want their son to look different from his father or other boys his age at school. The other reason is health related, including reducing urinary-tract infections (UTIs) in the first year of baby's life and reducing a man's chances of developing cancer or contracting syphilis or HIV in later life. The reduction in UTIs falls from 1 in a 100 for an uncircumcised male to 1 in 1,000 for a circumcised infant during baby's first year.

Most parents are concerned about the pain a child experiences with this procedure. The American Academy of Pediatrics (AAP) now states that pain relief is essential when a newborn is circumcised. Various techniques are available and recommended, including dorsal penile nerve block, the subcutaneous ring block or a topical anesthetic cream.

Risks with the procedure are minor and include some bleeding and local infection. The wound usually heals in about 10 days.

Should Our Baby Be Circumcised?

In the recent past, most infant boys were circumcised. Today, some parents are choosing not to have this surgical procedure performed on their baby. It's a personal decision.

The American Academy of Pediatrics has taken a neutral stand on circumcision. They have concluded there is no right or wrong answer to the question. The association believes the decision is up to the parents and is based on medical reasons and cultural and religious beliefs.

If you decide to have your son circumcised, performing the surgery at this early age will have little effect on him. (Postponing it until later years can be significantly more painful and carry higher risks.) If you decide not to have the procedure performed, your child will not be the only child who is uncircumcised as he grows up. Statistically, about 1/3 of his male friends and acquaintances will also be uncircumcised. Circumcision requires surgical permission from you and your partner; it won't be done without your consent.

When you meet with your pediatrician before baby's birth, circumcision may be a subject you want to cover. If you don't have that opportunity, you can always discuss it before baby leaves the hospital.

FEEDING YOUR BABY

The decision of how your partner will feed baby is one that most new fathers leave to the mother. After all, she's the one who will be involved with feeding the baby, so what kind of input can a father actually have? A lot, according to researchers.

Studies show that the most common reason a woman gives up breastfeeding her baby is the father's negative attitude. One report indicated that more than 75% of all men decide *before* pregnancy or during the *first trimester* whether they want their partner to breastfeed. One reason cited by the men is that they were afraid how society would view their partner if she breastfed in public. The good news is that when many of these men were made aware of the nutritional advantages and health benefits to baby that breastfeeding provides, they changed their attitudes and supported their partners.

Breast milk contains all the nutrients a baby needs, and it's easy for baby to digest. Breastfed babies have lower rates of infection because of the immunological content of breast milk. Breastfeeding can also give the baby a sense of security and the mother a sense of self-esteem. However, if there are reasons your partner cannot or chooses not to breastfeed, your baby will do well if you feed him or her formula.

IN THE DOGHOUSE

If your partner decides to breastfeed your baby, don't think about how she may appear to others. Most women can breastfeed discretely. Breastfeeding supplies your baby with the best start in life he or she can have!

Discuss breastfeeding with your partner during pregnancy. Support her in whatever she decides to do; you can be a big support and help with either choice. If she is breastfeeding, you can help out at night by getting up and bringing baby to her to nurse. If she's bottle-feeding, you can take over some of the feedings—you can even switch off for night feedings.

11

Now You're a Dad!

R ight now, you may be a little uncertain about what your "dad" role is and will be. Your partner may be taking care of baby while you sit on the sidelines, wondering what you can and should do. Our advice—get involved! Start immediately to be responsible for various aspects of caring for your baby. Once you get started, you'll quickly become a pro.

You may be uncertain about what things a new father is capable of doing. You can do just about anything—with the exception of breast-feeding your baby. You can even help out with that when the new mom expresses her breast milk; you can feed baby a bottle of it. Or you can get up at night and bring baby to mom. Other tasks you can easily handle include bathing baby, getting baby ready for bed, rocking and soothing your little one, changing diapers and helping mom.

In today's world, fathers are more involved than ever with their children. Studies show that dads now spend more time with their children than they did in the past. As recently as 1990, fathers only spent about 43% as much time with their kids as mothers did. Today, that figure is 65% as much time as moms during the week, and 87% as much as moms on the weekend. Much of the time is spent in child-care duties, which can help bring a father closer to his children. And it helps dad to feel more like a true parent, too.

NOTE. For the sake of clarity and understanding, in this chapter we use the term "him" when referring to baby in some sections; in the following section, we will use "her."

Chapter Focus

In this last chapter, we discuss life after pregnancy, as you begin your new lives together as a family. First we examine what it takes to be a good dad, followed by adjusting to life with your baby. Then we touch upon common concerns new fathers express, explore your "couple relationship," which may become even more important now that you and your partner have a child together, and finish with a discussion of postpartum distress syndrome, which can affect both your partner and you.

WHAT DOES IT TAKE TO BE A GOOD DAD?

Fatherhood is now upon you. The way you describe yourself has changed to add "dad" or "father" to your list of titles. Although you have changed, you still remain the same. You are just adding another wonderful job to your list of accomplishments.

Being a father carries great responsibility, and you probably want to do the best job you can. The role lasts forever—even when your children are grown and have children of their own (it's hard to imagine that it will ever happen with a new baby in your arms), you'll still be a dad. Knowing how to begin, and how to continue through the many years ahead, is a big help. Don't take a "wait and see" attitude—jump in with both feet! It's great on-the-job training, and you and baby will both learn as you go.

Don't be afraid to ask for help and guidance if you need it. No one is an expert immediately—not even your partner! And no one expects you to be, either! It doesn't diminish you in any way to ask others for direction. As a matter of fact, they will probably admire you for having the courage to know you need assistance and that you are confident enough to ask for it.

Talk to other parents, especially other fathers, about your concerns. Many have had the same experiences you are having. Their solutions to some of the problems you may worry about or experience can save you anxiety and hassles. Your increased feelings of confidence will help strengthen your attachment with your new baby.

"New Baby" Lingo

If you come across terms you don't understand when reading about your new baby or at a visit with the pediatrician, check the section "After Baby's Birth" in the *Pregnancy-Related Terms for Expecting Couples,* which begins on page 15. It contains some definitions of terms you may want to know.

Bonding with Baby

Women have 9 months to bond with their baby before it is born. Some experts believe you can also begin bonding with your baby before delivery. We discuss this in Chapter 5. Although it's important for a mother and baby to bond, it is equally important for a man to bond with his child. Bonding allows you to connect physically and emotionally with your baby. It usually doesn't happen instantly, and it isn't a one-time event. But it is one of the most important things you can do with your baby, and it helps you truly realize your baby is your own.

As a new father, you need time to bond with your newborn. You can continue this wonderful journey soon after baby's birth. It's important to spend time alone with your baby to strengthen your feelings of attachment. After baby is born, hold him close, gaze into his eyes and coo. Stroking and rubbing baby while making eye contact heightens the bonding effect. Babies readily respond to the human voice, so sing and talk to him to help strengthen the connection.

Bonding Techniques

There are many techniques you can use to bond with your baby. Some techniques that fathers have used include the following activities. Try those that you believe might work for you. Don't worry about appearing silly or foolish—no one but you and baby will know what you do!

✓ Lie on your side on the bed. Lay baby on his side facing you. Pull him close so he can feel your breath on his face. Sing or talk to him as you rub or stroke his body.

✓ Hold your baby so his head snuggles under your chin. (Be sure you have shaved recently so you don't give him whisker burn!) Sway from side to side, and coo or sing to him. He will feel your warm breath as you exhale.

✓ Lay baby on his stomach along your forearm. Support his head and chin with your hand. Let his legs hang down on either side of your arm. Carry him in this position, or sit in a chair together. Protect his head if you move around carrying him like this.

✓ Lie on the bed with your baby. Have your shirt off, and lay your naked (or diapered) baby against your bare skin. (This is one of the recommended bonding positions for moms as soon as baby is born.) Turn baby's head to the side so he can hear your heartbeat. Relax together, and enjoy the closeness.

✓ Keep baby close as you go through your day. Take baby with you on errands; "wear" baby in a snuggler on your chest. Hearing your voice, smelling your individual scent and being close to you will help both of you become closer.

✓ As baby grows older, keep in close contact by holding and/or hugging him. Physical contact with a son will *not* make him less masculine as he grows older. Showing your feelings is a great gift to give baby—and your bond will be strong.

✓ Performing the tasks of parenthood—feeding, changing, comforting baby—are terrific times to bond. It's OK for a dad to learn how to diaper, bathe and dress a baby! Help out whenever you can, and you and your baby will get to know each other even better.

POSITIVE ASPECTS OF BONDING.   There are many positive aspects for you and baby when you form a strong bond. Baby will be relaxed and comfortable with you. You will know how to care for baby when the opportunity arises. It's also physically healthy for you. Studies show that relaxing with your baby can help lower your heart rate and blood pressure. Bonding is good for you both!

Things to Do as You Embark on the "Fatherhood" Journey

There are many ways to move positively into fatherhood after baby arrives. Learn about child care; read our book *Your Baby's First Year Week by Week* and other books and articles about the many aspects of parenthood you may have questions about. Practice what you learn. It's good to be informed, but it doesn't help your partner or you or your baby if you don't try out what you're learning.

Many men have the false notion that a woman instinctively knows how to care for a baby. In some cases, this is true; in others, the woman hasn't a clue what to do. Don't wrongly assume that a new mother will be better able to handle the new-baby situation. You need to be as proactive as she is.

Below is a list of things many new fathers have shared with us that helped them start their journey down the parenting path. Read them over, discuss them with your partner and use what works for you as a family.

✓ Spend time with your partner and new baby. Don't bury yourself in work to escape what's going on at home. Both your partner and baby need your time and attention.

✓ Realize that each parent brings different resources to a situation. Decide who can do what, and share the responsibilities.

✓ Allow your partner time to herself, especially when she is home all day with baby. She needs a break, so tend baby while she relaxes. She can spend some quiet time by herself, get out of the house to see a friend or even just go grocery shopping.

✓ Let your partner know when you need some time to yourself, too. Doing something you enjoy, such as playing tennis, jogging or going bowling, can help you deal with stress.

✓ Attend pediatrician appointments, when you can. It's good to learn from an expert how your baby is doing. Suggestions can be made to both of you if changes might benefit your baby.

✓ Volunteer for some of the less glamorous baby chores, such as changing diapers, feeding baby at 2am or calming and comforting (hopefully!) a crying baby. You don't have to do these tasks all the time, but doing them some of the time will earn your partner's gratitude and appreciation.

✓ Acknowledge the job your partner is doing taking care of baby. It can be difficult to recover physically and emotionally from pregnancy while caring for an infant. It takes time, so offer her your support.

✓ Consider taking paternity leave. Staying home with baby, especially if you're the sole caregiver for that time, helps you bond with baby, appreciate your partner's efforts and become a better parent.

✓ Keep your emotions in check. It may be difficult to deal with your partner's mood swings after baby's birth (see the discussion on *Postpartum Distress Syndrome* that begins on page 257), but it will serve you well if you do. The problem will soon pass.

✓ You may feel depressed, too; it's normal for some men. If this happens to you, talk to your partner about it. Ask for her understanding, and try to work out a solution that is right for you both.

✓ If you don't know something, and you want to learn about it, observe and ask questions—of your partner, friends and professionals. Listen closely to what they say, and pay attention to details.

✓ Ask your partner for feedback on how you're doing. After all, you can't improve at a task unless you know *how* to improve!

✓ Trust your instincts. You have them, and your partner has them. You'll come to know your little one quite well and may instinctually know how to take care of something. If something doesn't seem right, it probably isn't.

✓ Now that baby is here, your friends and family members can be even more important than in the past. Don't cut yourselves off from other adults and adult activities and fun.

✓ Realize you can't prepare for everything. Be as prepared as you can be, then sit back and relax.

Some Specific Things You Should Know

Knowing some baby-care basics can really help you out when baby needs care. If you can do the following, you'll be in control most of the time. Then you can relax and enjoy your "job."

- *Know how to hold an infant.* Always support and protect baby's head. Hold baby in your arms, or put baby on your shoulder.

- *Learn what it takes to soothe your crying baby.* As you get to know baby better, you'll become experienced at what works with her.

- *Ask your partner or someone else to teach you how to bathe baby.* You can clean up baby when she needs it; it may also help soothe her when she's fussy.

- *Become an expert at feeding baby a bottle.* If your partner bottlefeeds, you can take over some of the feeding chores on a permanent basis. If she breastfeeds, you can feed baby a bottle of expressed milk whenever the need arises.

- *Establish and use a bedtime routine for baby.* It helps to know what to do when this important task falls on your shoulders. And it can help settle baby when she's cranky.

- *Take time to discover how to travel with baby.* Do it! (Small trips around town are good learning experiences.) Find out what you need when you go, and learn how to pack a diaper bag.

ADJUSTING TO LIFE WITH BABY

With a new baby in the house, your lives have suddenly changed! You and your partner will make many adjustments in the days, weeks, months and even years ahead. Some of the changes you make in your life now may have an impact for years to come. Other changes will work until your baby enters some new physical, emotional or developmental stage, then you'll have to make new adjustments. In this section, we address ways you can help make attuning your lives to baby's easier and more enjoyable.

You've looked forward for months to welcoming your new baby into your life. It's exciting to bond together as a family.

Baby's Schedule
Can Impact on His Parents
During your baby's first days and weeks at home, you may begin to wonder if all he will ever do is eat, sleep and wet or mess his diapers. You may wonder if he'll ever get on

> Be aware that mistakes will be made by you and your partner—every new parent makes them. But don't fret over a situation; learn from your error and move on.

any type of schedule. Let your baby develop his own schedule. You'll be able to make changes as he grows and develops.

You may find your baby sleeps a lot. It's also normal for a baby to get day and night mixed up for a while, but it doesn't usually last longer than a few weeks. If possible, keep baby awake and active during the day. It may help him get on a better sleep schedule.

In the first 4 weeks of life, baby may sleep as many as 20 hours a day. You may wonder if he will ever be awake long enough to get to know him. But he will soon be up more each day. When he is awake, cuddle and love him. Each day he will become more aware of you and his surroundings.

Get Enough Sleep and Rest
While your baby sleeps, it's important for both parents to try to get adequate rest. You probably won't be able to get 7 or 8 hours of

uninterrupted sleep, but you can take naps and go to bed earlier than usual to help reach that goal. Studies have shown that even a few days of sleep deprivation can increase a person's chances of becoming ill. You and your partner need to be in good health to take care of your baby.

One of the best things you can do is to sleep or rest when baby sleeps. Even if you are the primary caregiver at the time (maybe mom's resting or doing something that relaxes her), take a rest when baby's asleep.

If you can't sleep, that's OK. Just resting can help rejuvenate you. Lie down in bed or on the sofa, and let your mind drift.

Take Offers of Help

If you are fortunate enough to have family and friends around who want to help after baby comes home, let them! Many parents want to do everything by themselves, but when someone is willing to help out, it frees you to do other things. You may need to rest, or maybe you and your partner need to spend some adult time alone together.

If people ask how they can help, there are many things you can let them do. Ready-made meals to put in the refrigerator or freezer are always welcome. Cleaning services and laundry help are great gifts. You may be grateful if someone can watch the baby while you or your partner rest or take care of other tasks. When you let others help, you gain from it, and so do they.

Household Changes That Can Be Helpful

Keep the temperature in your home at a comfortable level. You don't need it too warm; when it is, it could be detrimental for *everyone* in the family. Generally, 68F (20C) to 70F (21C) is a good range. Baby's mood can be an indicator of how she's feeling. If you can't comfort your baby by holding or feeding her, she may be too hot or too cold.

Don't walk on tiptoes around your little one. Usual household noises won't harm baby; being exposed to them will make her less sensitive to them. You'll find she'll have an easier time sleeping (anywhere, not just at home) if she's used to background noises in your home.

PRECAUTIONS TO TAKE AT HOME. It's also important to take some precautions to make your house safe for baby. You may not think this is important when your baby is so small, but it is. There are many things you can do to help keep baby safe from the first day you bring him home.

No one can completely babyproof a house, but there are things you can do to make your home safer. Accidents can and do (and will!) happen, so to help prevent them, keep in mind the following.

✓ Crib slats should not be farther apart than 2⅜ inches (6cm)(you shouldn't be able to pass a soda can through the bars). The mattress should fit securely. Don't put *anything* in the crib but a fitted crib sheet and baby (to help reduce the risk of sudden-infant-death syndrome).

✓ Keep the crib's dropside up and locked when baby is in it.

✓ Keep mobiles and other crib toys out of baby's reach. You may have to remove them as baby grows older.

✓ Keep the crib away from windows, wall decorations, heating units, climbable furniture, blind cords, drapery pulls and other possible dangers.

✓ Never hang a pacifier or any other object around baby's neck.

✓ Never leave a baby alone in the water, even if it's only a few inches deep. A baby can drown in as little as 1 inch of water, and it only takes a minute!

✓ Never leave baby unattended on a sofa, chair, changing table or any other surface above the floor. He could easily roll off.

✓ Never put an infant seat on the counter or a table while baby is in it.

✓ Always use safety straps with baby equipment.

✓ Follow directions for using all baby equipment. The manufacturer provides them for the safety of your baby.

✓ Never hold or carry your baby while you're cooking, drinking a hot beverage or smoking a cigarette.

✓ If you warm formula or heat baby food in the microwave, shake the bottle or stir the food before serving to avoid hot spots. Don't heat breast milk in the microwave—it changes the immunological properties of the milk.

✓ Don't hang anything on stroller handles; the extra weight could cause the stroller to tip over.

✓ *Always* put your baby in a car seat. Be sure the car seat meets federal safety guidelines and is properly installed. Sign up for any recalls so you will be notified if something comes up later.

✓ Keep stairs and other areas well lit.

✓ Use nonslip mats in the tub and on the bathroom floor to help prevent falls.

✓ Install antiscald devices in tubs and showers.

COMMON CONCERNS FOR NEW FATHERS

Most new fathers have various concerns about how their lives will change now that baby is here. Having a baby doesn't have to be the end of your life as you knew it "before baby." You have probably made many adjustments during your life to deal with changes. This is just another opportunity to grow and to learn. In fact, you may find that changes you make now may improve your life as a family man. Some men discover the best times they have are those spent with their new baby and their partner.

AM I READY TO BE A DAD? If you ask most first-time parents, and they give you an honest answer, probably *none* of them felt they were ready for this new direction in their lives. Why? One reason is fear of the unknown. As parents ourselves, we know for a fact that no one can tell you what it's like to be a parent. Along this same line, you can't know the joy that comes with being a parent until you experience it for yourself. So accept your anxiety as a common emotion many new parents have.

Once you have experienced what is expected of you as a father, your unease will probably vanish. Just *being* a parent may take away a great deal of your worry. When you're involved in doing the job, it won't seem so difficult, and you'll discover the joys of being a dad.

CAN I CARE FOR BABY? Many men fear they will be unable to care for a baby; often baby care is portrayed as something men can't do. One of the best ways to deal with this concern is to get some on-the-job training. Practical experience is the best way to learn. In child-birth-education classes, you may learn how to diaper and bathe a baby. If you have friends or family members with a new baby, offer your babysitting expertise as a couple for a day or evening, and try out your skills. It might also be good for the mom-to-be to practice.

OUR COUPLE RELATIONSHIP WILL NEVER BE THE SAME. In a way, you're right. Your relationship has probably changed forever, but that can be a good thing. Now you are partners in parenting, as well as in life, and your relationship will change to reflect the many adjustments and adaptations you are both making.

You both need to work on the positive aspects of being a couple. See the discussion of *Your Couple Relationship* below.

YOUR COUPLE RELATIONSHIP

With baby part of your family now, you may be wondering how this will affect your relationship with your partner. Will you be as close as you once were? Will you ever have sex again? How can you keep the flame of your passion burning?

You need to be realistic about what has happened to you. You have become parents, so that is one very important aspect of your relationship. But you are also a couple—you were a couple *before* baby's birth, and you probably want to preserve the meaningful relationship you shared then. It takes work to do this. You both need to be committed to maintaining and preserving the connection you share. In this section, we will share some ideas with you that have worked for many other couples in the same situation.

Be Considerate of Each Other, and Treat Yourselves Well
After the months of pregnancy and the stress of adjusting to life with a new baby, you may wonder if you'll ever get back into the swing of

things as a couple. Planning on your part to handle the demands on your time and energies can help. Rewarding yourselves occasionally is also beneficial.

What You May Learn from Your Baby

You may be wondering what an infant who cannot hold his head up or roll over can teach you. You may be surprised by how much you will discover from this little fellow, if you take the time to learn. Parenting will teach you many things, if you are a willing student.

Some of the things parents have told us they learned from their babies include the following.

- *Slow down.* You've probably heard the adage, "Stop and smell the roses." You can't stop and smell the roses if you don't slow down first. With your new baby, take the time to appreciate what life has given you. Live in the moment. Put aside (for a while) worries about work deadlines, household chores and finances. Enjoy what's happening now!

- *Don't try to be perfect.* Once baby is on the scene, perfection goes out the window. We're not saying you can't be focused and do your best when you do something. What we're saying is that perfection is unnecessary. You can't be perfect; you're wasting your time, energy and talents if you try to be. Your life shouldn't be perfect, either. That leaves no room for making changes and adjustments when they are necessary. And no baby is perfect—it's a fact—nor should they be. Babies learn from making mistakes. So relax and enjoy your life for the growth and transformations you are all experiencing.

- *Keep trying, even when it seems impossible.* A baby learns to master a task by trying it over and over and over again. When he fails, he keeps trying because each time he tries to do something and fails, he learns from the experience. We can do the same thing. The old saying, "Failure only means you tried" certainly applies to baby's efforts. Maybe it can apply to your efforts, too.

Think about ways you can pamper yourself and your partner. The following suggestions may help you make your lives together more enjoyable.

GIVE EACH OTHER SOME SPACE.   You'll soon discover how valuable it is for each of you to have some quiet time to yourself. You may enjoy working on a project, doing some research on the computer or playing a game of golf. Your partner may enjoy a long soak in the tub or spending time alone reading or doing crafts. When you each have some time alone, it helps you renew your inner strength and your commitment to your couple relationship.

PAMPER EACH OTHER.   Do something special for each other or yourselves as a couple when you can. Eat a romantic dinner at home together. Or hire a babysitter or ask friends or family members to take care of baby while the two of you go to a movie, a play or a concert. A couple of hours together gives you adult time to renew your relationship.

**MEMORABLE MOMENTS
FROM DR. DAD**

As I was doing rounds, seeing patients who had just delivered babies, I met Kay and Bob getting ready to leave the hospital with their new baby girl. Bob had the baby securely snuggled in his arms, with a tired but happy expression on his face. He was looking lovingly at his daughter. He looked up in surprise when I said hello to him. He had been so absorbed in the baby that he hadn't even seen me. I asked Kay how she was doing, and she said she was well and pleasantly surprised at how quickly Bob had bonded with their baby. He was protective and possessive of the baby, which was a change of attitude because he had not been that involved during the pregnancy. Bob related to me the flood of emotions and joy he felt growing inside him as he took on the new role of fatherhood.

MASSAGE IS GOOD FOR BOTH OF YOU.   If you practiced massage techniques during pregnancy, use some of that expertise now to help each other relax. If you don't know anything about massage, there are some excellent books and videos available to check out at the library or to rent or buy at a video store that provide instructions on "couple massage." We're not talking about anything sexual; the techniques we recommend are for relaxation and stress reduction.

DEAL WITH YOUR FEELINGS.   It's important for your relationship for both of you to deal effectively with your feelings. The three "Cs" are important in this process—*communication, compromise* and *cooperation.*

When a difficult situation arises, begin by expressing your feelings. Be specific, and encourage your partner to do the same. Open communication can help you both. Discuss issues as they arise so you can deal with them, and be honest about your feelings and concerns. Then compromise about the solution (if it's necessary), and cooperate together in putting the plan into action.

My Mother-in-Law Said

If you pick up baby every time she cries, you'll spoil her.

The truth is you *should* pick up baby whenever she cries, especially in the first few months of life. This helps baby feel secure in the awareness that you'll be there in times of distress, when she is uncomfortable or scared, or whenever she needs you. Picking up and comforting a crying baby is the *right* thing to do!

Will We Have Sex Again?

Probably one of the most important things on your mind right now is resuming sexual relations. Most men are eager for this aspect of their couple relationship to begin again. However, many women express the feeling that sex at this time is too painful and too much to cope with. They need to rest, get enough sleep and get back into a routine before they start thinking about sex again.

Resuming sexual relations can be a little difficult. In the past, we advised a woman to wait at least 6 weeks before having intercourse. Today, we tell a woman to let her body be her guide, but 6 weeks is still a good suggestion. Don't expect to resume relations with your partner 1 or 2 weeks after delivery. Don't press her; let her resume sexual intercourse when she feels ready. When you do begin sharing this important aspect of your lives again together, take it easy and go slowly. Encourage your partner to share her feelings and concerns with you.

Your partner's sex drive can be affected by stress, emotions and fatigue. Your sex drive may be affected by many of the same things, as well.

DON'T FORGET ABOUT BIRTH CONTROL.   When you begin having intercourse, take precautions if you don't want another pregnancy immediately. Your partner can become pregnant *before* she has a menstrual period. It's important for her to discuss birth-control options with you and her doctor, either in the hospital or at her 6-week postpartum checkup.

Working Together as Parents

If you begin your role as parents by working together, you'll probably accomplish a great deal. Dividing parenting duties and responsibilities as evenly as possible between the two of you may make it easier for you both to parent your baby. Parenting takes a lot of hard work, and it can be very stressful. But the rewards are great. Working together to create a team with your partner can increase those rewards.

The fact that there are two of you will naturally introduce differences on the way some tasks should be handled, but this can be beneficial. Make an attempt to work together—not at odds with each other—to provide consistency

BROWNIE POINTS

Teaching values is a difficult task. The best way to do it is to set an example. Always strive to be a good role model for your child.

IN THE DOGHOUSE

Don't expect your partner to "be the parent." You need to play an active role in your child's life, right from the start. If you don't, you may find it hard later to become a part of her life.

in your child's life. Agree in the beginning that it's OK for each of you to have different ways of doing things, but that you will be consistent in whatever you do.

One of the most common areas of concern is disagreements—it will be impossible for you and your partner to agree on everything. It may help to understand that each of you brings to this parenting relationship your own background of feelings and thoughts. You each may have a different "take" on a situation. This can create problems if you don't set up ways in advance to deal with the differences. Discuss your expectations *before* baby's birth. It's easier to find out what your partner believes before you each get caught up in the stress of parenting. You may be surprised (pleasantly or not) at what your partner believes each parental role should be.

IN THE DOGHOUSE

Don't always say "Yes"; learn to say "No" to your child. Although you'll probably find it easier as your child gets older to say "Yes," a good parent knows when to say "No."

Share duties. If you are both experienced in all facets of caring for your baby, you'll be able to handle change more easily.

Stay flexible. Different people have different ways of doing things that bring about the same results. There are usually many solutions at hand—be open to doing things a different way. It may save you time and effort to accept the "different" way your partner does something.

Support each other, even if you have different opinions. Talk about your different takes on a situation, and work to resolve it.

Work toward an emotional balance. Support each other in your efforts to be good parents.

Consider each other's perspective. When a situation arises that you disagree on, try to see it from the other's point of view. Sometimes this shift in perspective can be very beneficial to you both.

POSTPARTUM DISTRESS SYNDROME

In the recent past, there has been a great deal of media coverage of postpartum depression; discussion of the problem in its entirety is called *postpartum distress syndrome*. Most people don't understand what it is; many dismiss it as a "minor problem." Most of the time it *is* a minor problem, and it can be dealt with fairly easily. Occasionally, it is more serious.

Many women experience some degree of postpartum distress; in fact, up to 80% of all women get the "baby blues" within a short time after their baby's birth. Baby blues usually appear between 2 days and 2 weeks after a baby is born. The good news is that the situation is temporary and tends to leave as quickly as it comes.

Today, many medical experts consider some degree of postpartum distress normal. Symptoms include anxiety, lack of confidence, crying for no reason, lack of feeling for the baby, exhaustion, low self-esteem, impatience, oversensitivity, irritability and restlessness. At this time, we are not sure what causes postpartum distress. We believe a woman's individual sensitivity to hormonal changes may be part of the cause.

If you believe your partner may be suffering from some form of postpartum distress, contact the doctor. Every postpartum reaction, mild or severe, is usually temporary.

BROWNIE POINTS

Show your child you love him by being a steady, reliable influence in his life. There is no substitution for your love, attention and presence in your child's life.

Forms of Postpartum Distress
The mildest form of postpartum distress is called the *baby blues*.

The problem lasts only a couple of weeks, and symptoms do not worsen.

A more serious version of postpartum distress is called *postpartum depression* (PPD); it affects about 10% of all new mothers. The difference between baby blues and postpartum depression lies in the frequency, intensity and duration of symptoms. Sleep problems are one way to distinguish between the two. If the mother can sleep while someone else tends her baby, it is probably baby blues. If she cannot sleep because of anxiety, it's probably PPD.

PPD can occur from 2 weeks to 1 year after birth. A mother may have feelings of anger, confusion, panic and hopelessness, and may experience changes in her eating and sleeping patterns. She may fear she will hurt her baby or feel as if she is going crazy. Anxiety is one of the major symptoms of PPD.

The most serious form of postpartum distress is *postpartum psychosis*. The woman may have hallucinations, think about suicide or try to harm the baby.

Dealing with the Problem

One of the most important ways to help your partner deal with the problem is to set up a support system before baby's birth. Ask family members and friends to help. Have your mother or mother-in-law stay for a while. You might be able to take some leave from work to help out at home. If you can't, you might consider hiring someone to come in and help each day.

There is no one specific treatment for baby blues, but there are ways you can help relieve your partner's symptoms. Ask for help from others. Encourage the new mom to rest when baby sleeps. Help her find other mothers who are in the same situation; it can help her to share her feelings and experiences. Let her know it's OK not to be perfect. Pamper her. Support her in her efforts to do some form of moderate exercise every day. Oversee the menu so you both eat nutritiously. Motivate her to go out every day.

Go with your partner to an office visit with the doctor if her experience goes beyond baby blues. At your visit, discuss what actions you might take. With postpartum depression, medication may be necessary. About 85% of all women who suffer from postpartum depression require medication. Medications of choice include antidepressants, tranquilizers and hormones; often they are used together.

Postpartum Distress Can Also Affect You

You can be affected if your partner suffers from the baby blues or PPD. A recent study found that about 3% of all new fathers experience significant depression following their partner's pregnancy. The study also showed that when a new mom feels depressed, her partner's chance of being depressed increases significantly.

It's important to prepare yourself for this situation. Understand that if you or your partner become depressed, it's only temporary. Other things you can do to help yourself include the following.

✓ Get professional help if you need it. It isn't a sign of weakness; it's a sign of strength and maturity.

✓ Don't take your partner's situation personally.

✓ Get support from friends, family members and other fathers.

✓ Take care of yourself by eating well, getting enough rest and exercising.

✓ Be patient with your partner.

✓ Give her your love and support during this difficult time. Ask her to do the same for you.

Good Luck to You All!

We hope the information in this book has been helpful to you and your partner as you have moved through pregnancy, experienced the birth of your baby and begun life as a family. We know from experience that the most wonderful times of your life lie ahead of you.

We wish you luck as you grow together as a family. You may go through many surprising experiences as your child (or children) grow. Open yourself to these opportunities for growth, and enjoy each and every day. You are truly blessed to be able to take on the role of "Dad."

Resources

GENERAL INFORMATION FOR PARENTS

For Adoptive Parents
Good resource for adoption information
www.adoption.com

American Academy of Pediatrics (AAP)
P.O. Box 927, Dept. C
Elk Grove Village, IL 60009-0927
www.aap.org

American Academy of Family Practitioners (AAFP)
www.aafp.com

American College of Obstetricians and Gynecologists (ACOG)
P.O. Box 4500
Kearneysville, WV 25430
800-762-2264
www.acog.com

American Psychological Association (APA)
202-336-5700
www.apa.org

Baby Doppler
To buy a home-use doppler to hear baby's heartbeat at home
888-758-8822
www.babybeat.com

Birth-Marker
Product for marking infant in hospital so baby mix-ups don't occur
www.birth-mark.com

California Cryobank Cord Blood Services
For information on storing baby's umbilical-cord blood
www.cryobank.com/baby

Car-Seat Installation
877-FIT-4-A-KID
www.fitforakid.com

Centers for Disease Control and Prevention
For up-to-date information on many medical issues
www.cdc.gov

Child Care Aware
800-424-2246

Children's Defense Fund
www.childrensdefense.org

COPE
37 Clarendon St.
Boston, MA 02116
617-357-5588

Home Testing for Pregnancy
Compares various pregnancy tests
www.kerouac.pharm.uky.edu/hometests/pregnancy/ptoc.html

Intensive-Care Parenting magazine
ICU Parenting
RD #10, Box 176
Brush Creek Rd.
Irwin, PA 15642

Internal Revenue Service
For information on child-care expenses
800-829-1040
www.irs.ustreas.gov

Juvenile Products Manufacturers Association (JPMA)
For information on baby products, recalls and other pertinent information
236 Route 38 West, Suite 100
Moorestown, NJ 08057
www.jpma.org

March of Dimes
For information on various tests before and during pregnancy
888-663-4637
www.modimes.org

Military Families
For families of military personnel
www.4militaryparents.com

National Organization of Single Mothers
P.O. Box 68
Midland, NC 28107-0068
704-888-KIDS (704-888-5437)

On-line announcements
Send on-line announcements and invitations for every occasion
www.senada.com
www.growingfamily.com

Parent's Resources
P.O. Box 107, Planetarium Sta.
New York, NY 10024
212-866-4776

Product Recalls
For the latest baby-product recalls and warnings
www.childrecall.com
www.cpsc.gov
www.jpma.org

Sidelines
For women experiencing complicated pregnancies
Candace Hurley, executive director: 714-497-2265
Tracy Hoogenboom: 909-563-6199

Social Security Administration
800-772-1213
www.ssa.gov

Spina Bifida Association of America
For information on various tests before and during pregnancy
800-623-141
www.sbaa.org

U.S. Consumer Products Safety Commission (CPSC)
800-638-2772
www.cpsc.gov

U.S. Department of Agriculture (USDA)
For information on the food pyramid
www.cnpp.usda.gov

Vaccines
For information on vaccines from the Children's Hospital of Philadelphia
www.vaccine.chop.edu

Virtual Birth Center
By state, lists obstetricians, midwives, birth centers, doulas and other services
www.virtualbirth.com

The Women's Bureau Publications
For summary of state laws on family leave
U.S. Department of Labor
Women's Bureau Clearing House
Box EX
200 Constitution Avenue, NW
Washington, D.C. 20210
800-827-5335
Also see www.ecoc.gov/facts/fs-preg.html

Websites for further information
www.americanbaby.com
www.babycenter.com
www.babyzone.com
www.bellycast.com
www.childmagazine.com
www.ibaby.com
www.ivillage.com
www.parenthoodweb.com

AT-HOME MOMS

F.E.M.A.L.E. (Formerly Employed Mothers At The Leading Edge)
P.O. Box 31
Elmhurst, IL 60126
800-223-9399
www.femalehome.org

Miserly Moms
Helps families save money by providing tips for cooking, shopping, decorating and gardening
www.miserlymoms.com

Mothers At Home
800-783-4666
www.mah.org

MOMS (Mothers Offering Mothers Support)
25371 Rye Canyon Rd.
Valencia, CA 91355
805-526-2725

Websites for further information
www.momsonline.com
www.parentsplace.com
www.parentssoup.com
www.parenttime.com

BREASTFEEDING INFORMATION

Avent
800-542-8368
www.aventamerica.com

Best Start
3500 E. Fletcher Avenue, Suite 519
Tampa, FL 33613
800-277-4975

Breastfeeding Basics
www.breastfeedingbasics.com

Breastfeeding Help
For 24-hour breastfeeding support, referrals to lactation consultants and helpful videos
www.breastfeeding.com

Food and Drug Administration (FDA) Hotline
800-332-4010

FDA Breast Implant Information Line
800-532-4440

International Lactation Consultant Association
919-787-5181

La Leche League International
1400 North Meacham Road
Schaumburg, IL 60173-4840
800-LA-LECHE or check local telephone directory
www.lalecheleague.org

Medela, Inc.
P.O. Box 660
McHenry, IL 60051
800-TELL-YOU (800-735-5968)

National Center for Nutrition and Dietetics; Consumer Nutrition Hotline
800-366-1655

National Maternal and Child Health Clearinghouse
2070 Chain Bridge Road, Suite 45
Vienna, VA 22182
703-821-8955, ext. 254

Wellstart
4062 First Avenue
San Diego, CA 92103
619-295-5192

Websites for further information
www.moms4milk.org
www.breastfeed.com

CHILDBIRTH INFORMATION

American Academy of Husband-Coached Childbirth
(Bradley Method)
P.O. Box 5224
Sherman Oaks, CA 91413
800-422-4784; 818-788-6662

American College of Nurse-Midwives (ACNM)
818 Connecticut Avenue, NW, Suite 900
Washington, D.C. 20006
202-728-9860

American Society for Psychoprophylaxis in Obstetrics (ASPO/Lamaze)
1200 19th Street, NW, Suite 300
Washington, D.C. 20036-2422
800-368-4404

Association of Labor Assistants and Childbirth Educators (ALACE)
P.O. Box 382724
Cambridge, MA 02238-2724
617-441-2500

Birth Centers
Lists birthing centers in 37 states
www.birthcenters.org

Doulas of North America
1100 23rd Avenue East
Seattle, WA 98112
FAX 206-325-0472
www.dona.com

Informed Home Birth
313-662-6852

International Cesarean Awareness Network (ICAN)
1304 Kingsdale Avenue
Redondo Beach, CA 90278
310-542-6400

International Childbirth Education Association
P.O. Box 20048
Minneapolis, MN 55420-0048
612-854-8660
Lamaze, *See American Society for Psychoprophylaxis in Obstetrics*
(above)

Midwives Alliance of North America (MANA)
P.O. Box 175
Newton, KS 67114
316-283-4543

National Association of Childbearing Centers (NACC)
3123 Gottschall Road
Perkiomenville, PA 18074
215-234-8068

Public Citizen's Health Research
For information on C-sections and VBAC
1600 20th Street, NW
Washington, D.C. 20009

CHILD CARE

Child Care Aware Hotline
800-424-2246

Department of Health and Human Services; National Child Care
Information Center
800-616-2242

International Nanny Association
800-297-1477
www.nanny.org

National Association of Child Care Resource and Referral Agencies
800-424-2246; 202-393-5501
www.childcarerr.org
www.naccrra.net

National Resource Center for Health and Safety in Child Care
800-598-5437
www.nrc.uchsc.edu

National Association for the Education of Young Children
www.naeyc.org

Working Mother
www.workingmother.com

DADS

At-Home Dad newsletter
61 Brightwood Ave.
North Andover, MA 01845
www.athomedad.com

Dad to Dad Network
Send self-addressed stamped envelope to:
13925 Duluth Court
Apple Valley, MN 55124
612-423-3705

Full-Time Dads
193 Shelley Ave.
Elizabeth, NJ 07208
908-355-9722
FAX 908-355-9723
www.fathersworld.com/fulltimedad

The Single & Custodial Father's Network
For fathers who are primary caregivers, to connect with other fathers in similar situations
www.single-fathers.org

Websites for further information
www.babycenter.com/dads
www.daddyshome.com
www.edads.com
www.fathersforum.com
www.fathersonline.com
www.fathersworld.com
www.manslife.com
www.newdads.com
www.portage.net/~rborelli/dads.html

FINANCIAL RESOURCES

BankRate
For general financial information
516-627-7330
www.bankrate.com

College Savings Plan Network
For information on saving for college
877-277-6496
www.savingforcollege.com

Consumer Credit Counseling Service
For help with your budget
888-775-0377

Consumer Federation of America
For information on many consumer situations
202-387-6121
www.consumerfed.org

Debtors Anonymous
For debt-management services
781-453-2743
www.debtorsanonymous.com

Easy Saver Plan
For information on government savings bonds and how to buy them
www.publicdebt.treas.gov

Health Insurance Association of America
For information on health and disability insurance
888-869-4078
www.hiaa.org

Insurance Information Institute
For information on various types of insurance
800-331-9146
www.iii.org

IntelliQuote Insurance Services
For quotes to compare for various insurance policies
888-622-0925
www.intelliquote.com

Internal Revenue Service (IRS)
For information on child-care expenses
800-829-1040
www.irs.ustreas.gov

National Association of Personal Planners
For help with your budget
888-333-6659

National Foundation for Credit Counseling
For debt-management services
800-388-2227
www.nfcc.org

National Insurance Consumer Helpline
For answers to specific insurance questions
800-942-4242

QuickQuote
For a term life insurance quote
800-867-2402
www.quickquote.com

Quotesmith
800-431-1147
www.quotesmith.com

U.S. Savings Bonds
800-4US-BONDS
www.savingsbonds.gov

Websites for further information
www.collegesavings.org
www.educationira.com
www.financenter.com
www.healthinsurancefinders.com
www.ihatefinancialplanning.com
www.insurance.com
www.localinsurance.com
www.mfea.com
www.morningstar.com
www.myvesta.org
www.naic.org/consumer.htm

MOTHER'S HEALTH

All About Kegels
Learn how to do Kegel exercises correctly
www.niddk.nih.gov/health/urolog/uibcw/exerc/exerc.htm
American Cancer Society
For information on the dangers of passive smoke
800-ACS-2345

Chiropractic Care
Discusses chiropractic care during pregnancy
www.rlx.net/babycottage/pregnancy.htm

Depression after Delivery
P.O. Box 1282
Morrisville, PA 19067
800-944-4773 (answering machine only)

Group-B Strep Association
P.O. Box 16515
Chapel Hill, NC 27516
919-932-5344

Mom's Fitness
For information and exercises to help pregnant women and new moms
www.fitmommies.com/pregnancy

Older Mothers-to-Be
For information for older expectant mothers
www.midlifemommies.com

Postpartum Support International
For information and help with postpartum distress syndrome
805-967-7636
www.postpartum.net

Preggie Pops
To help relieve morning sickness
www.preggiepops.com

Sideline (for women on bed rest)
714-497-2265

SOS Morning Sickness
For information on, and remedies for, nausea and vomiting
www.sosmorningsickness.com

MULTIPLES

Center for Loss in Multiple Birth
c/o Jean Kollantai
P.O. Box 1064
Palmer, AK 99645
907-746-6123

Center for Study of Multiple Births
333 E. Superior Street, Room 464
Chicago, IL 60611
312-266-9093

Mothers of Supertwins (M.O.S.T.) *(triplets or more)*
P.O. Box 951
Brentwood, NY 11717
516-434-MOST
www.mostonline.org

Multiple Birth Resources
70 W. Sylvester Place
Highland Ranch, CO 80126
888-627-9519
www.expectingmultiples.com

Multiple Births Foundation
Queen Charlotte's and Chelsea Hospital
Goldhawk Road
London, England WC2B OXG
081-748-4666, ext. 5201

National Online Fathers of Twins Club
www.member.aol.com/nofotc

National Organization of Mothers of Twins Clubs, Inc.
P.O. Box 438
Thompson Station, TN 37179-0438
505-275-0955

Triplet Connection
P.O. Box 99571
Stockton, CA 95209
209-474-0885
www.tripletconnection.org

Twin to Twin Transfusion Syndrome (TTTS) Foundation
Mary Slaman-Forsythe, Executive Director
411 Longbeach Parkway
Bay Village, OH 44140
216-899-8887

Twin Services
P.O. Box 10066
Berkeley, CA 94709
510-524-0863

The Twins Foundation
P.O. Box 6043
Providence, RI 02940-6043
401-729-1000

Twins Hope
International center for twin-related diseases
www.twinshope.com

Twins Magazine
5350 S. Roslyn Street, Suite 400
Englewood, CO 80111
800-328-3211

Twins World
Good resource for couples expecting multiples
www.twinsworld.com

NUTRITION INFORMATION

Beechnut Nutrition Hotline
800-523-6633

FDA Hotline
For nutrition information
800-332-4010

Food Guide Pyramid Brochure
USDA
P.O. Box 1144
Rockville, MD 20850
www.cnpp.usda.gov

PREMATURE INFANTS

ECMO Moms and Dads
c/o Blair and Gayle Wilson
P.O. Box 53848
Lubbock, TX 79453
806-794-0259

Intensive-Care Parenting magazine
ICU Parenting
RD #10, Box 176
Brush Creek Road
Irwin, PA 15642

Premature Babies
For information on, and products for, premature infants
www.earlyarrivals.com

SAFETY FOR YOUR BABY

Auto Safety Hotline
888-327-4236

Back to Sleep
P.O. Box 29111
Washington, D.C. 20040
800-505-2742

The Danny Foundation
For information on crib dangers
3158 Danville Blvd.
P.O. Box 680
Alamo, CA 94507
800-833-2669

General Motors
"Precious Cargo: Protecting the Children Who Ride with You" (free booklet)
800-247-9168

International Association of Chiefs of Police
Operation Kids
800-843-4227

Juvenile Products Manufacturers Association (JPMA)
236 Route 38 West, Suite 100
Moorestown, NJ 08057
www.jpma.org

National Highway Traffic Safety Administration (NHTSA)
800-424-99393
www.nhtsa.dot.gov

National Lead Information Hotline and Clearinghouse
800-424-LEAD

The National SAFE KIDS Campaign
800-441-1888
www.safekids.org

Nissan's Quest for Safety Campaign
"Car Seat Safety" (free booklet)
800-955-4500

Safety Alerts
For information on recalls
www.safetyalerts.com

SafetyBeltUSA
123 Manchester Blvd.
Inglewood, CA 90301
310-673-2666
www.carseat.org

U.S. Consumer Products Safety Commission
800-638-2772
www.cpsc.gov

Acknowledgments

There are many people we wish to thank for their help and support during the preparation of this book. Without their understanding and assistance, it would have been a harder task. We appreciate the help from the fathers and fathers-to-be who gave us their valuable insights, especially Lee Shreeve, Chris Rucinski, Scott Harbertson, Dave Stevens and Matthew Kilgore, and their wives (whom they supported during *their* pregnancies) Trish Shreeve, Heather Larson, Megan Harbertson, Kate Stevens and Patrizia Kilgore. Thanks also to David Cohen, CPA, Senior Partner, Beach, Fleischman & Co., P.C., Tucson, Arizona, for his valuable help with the financial information.

Glade Curtis, M.D.—My thanks to the many women and their partners over the years with whom I have had the privilege of sharing their pregnancy and childbirth. I've seen many men take an active part in their pregnancies, making a significant difference. They have been a valuable support and participant in the miracle of childbirth. As a father, and now as a grandfather, I marvel in the creation of families. Thanks to my wife, Debbie, our family and my parents for their endless love and support. Special thanks also to Scott and Megan Harbertson for financial expertise and computer skills.

Judith Schuler, M.S.—As always, thanks to my son, Ian, for your understanding and acceptance of everything that goes into writing a book. You've been through this process nine times now. And I greatly appreciate the continued love and support of my parents, Bob and Kay Gordon. Also, my gratitude to Bob Rucinski for your insights and valuable help with so many things related to preparing this book.

Index